Trauma and Crisis Counseling

Trauma and Crisis Counseling: An Overview for Emerging Professionals is an introduction to trauma for students, new counselors, and other helping professionals. The book provides a sweeping overview of trauma from more than 500 sources. It includes definitions, a clear exploration of trauma's neurobiology, information on assessment and diagnosis, and summaries of the primary models of evidence-based treatments. The text also addresses suicidality, crisis, and disasters, as well as the challenges faced in providing care to people who experience trauma. Throughout the book, the authors focus on what it means to be trauma-informed and how to integrate resiliency in trauma work. The material is presented in a conversational way using case studies, examples, and practical activities to enhance the reader's learning. *Trauma and Crisis Counseling* lays the foundation for effective trauma work in a readable format.

Kathy B. Hoppe, EdD, is an associate professor at Oral Roberts University and a licensed marriage and family therapist.

Michelle K. Taylor, EdD, is the director of the Master of Science in community counseling program at Rogers State University.

"Today's counselors are faced with a growing number of traumatized clients who need support and intervention. In this book, Hoppe and Taylor present the fundamentals counselors need to properly intervene. From the broad definition of the term 'trauma' to an explanation of trauma's significant impact, this book offers insight on the complexities of trauma intervention."

Kathy McDonald, PhD, associate professor and director of school counseling,
Southeastern Oklahoma State University

"This remarkably well-written book offers perspective and hope, emphasizing the critical importance of treating each trauma survivor as a unique individual rather than just a diagnosis. Highlighting the profound impact of a strong helper-client bond in increasing resilience and fostering hope underscores the transformative power of a compassionate approach. Educators and professionals alike will find this book an invaluable resource for understanding and supporting those who have experienced trauma."

Kim Haar, LPC, LMFT, CEO of There's Hope Counseling
and co-host on the Oasis Radio Network

"This is an invaluable tool for the field. As one who has been in victim services for over twenty-five years, the observations set forth in this text ring extraordinarily true. The resources and practice tips provided will help create a more enlightened, trauma-informed cadre of professionals who are better prepared to provide care for their clients and for themselves as they embark on this noble and demanding endeavor."

Sheree L. Hukill, MS, JD, victim services provider, administrator,
and visionary

Trauma and Crisis Counseling
An Overview for Emerging Professionals

Kathy B. Hoppe and Michelle K. Taylor

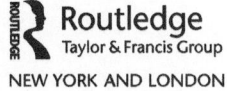
Routledge
Taylor & Francis Group

NEW YORK AND LONDON

Designed cover image: © Getty Images

First published 2025
by Routledge
605 Third Avenue, New York, NY 10158

and by Routledge
4 Park Square, Milton Park, Abingdon, Oxon, OX14 4RN

Routledge is an imprint of the Taylor & Francis Group, an informa business

Library of Congress Cataloging-in-Publication Data
Names: Hoppe, Kathy B., author. | Taylor, Michelle K., author.
Title: Trauma and crisis counseling : an overview for emerging
professionals / Kathy B. Hoppe and Michelle K. Taylor.
Description: New York, NY : Routledge, 2025. | Includes bibliographical
references and index.
Identifiers: LCCN 2024042301 (print) | LCCN 2024042302 (ebook) |
ISBN 9781032803548 (hardback) | ISBN 9781032803524 (paperback) |
ISBN 9781003496557 (ebook)
Subjects: LCSH: Psychic trauma--Patients--Counseling of. |
Psychic trauma--Treatment. | Counseling psychology.
Classification: LCC RC552.T7 H67 2025 (print) | LCC RC552.T7 (ebook) |
DDC 616.85/21--dc23/eng/20241122
LC record available at https://lccn.loc.gov/2024042301
LC ebook record available at https://lccn.loc.gov/2024042302

ISBN: 978-1-032-80354-8 (hbk)
ISBN: 978-1-032-80352-4 (pbk)
ISBN: 978-1-003-49655-7 (ebk)

DOI: 10.4324/9781003463009

Typeset in Univers
by SPi Technologies India Pvt Ltd (Straive)

Contents

Preface

We have a new graduate counseling program to address the increasing demand for mental health professionals. Should students pursue that path, the program meets the academic requirements for becoming a licensed professional counselor. We continually seek feedback from students, faculty, mental health professionals, and regional educators. Through a grounded theory framework, we identify gaps in the educational process in our program and across the region. Students overwhelmingly request practical courses focusing on trauma-informed care. As a result, we offer two trauma courses, the first covering a trauma overview, assessment, and evidence-based treatments, and the second focusing on somatic approaches. Our goal is to provide research-based courses that prepare students for real-world practice. By incorporating student feedback within a constructivist learning framework, we aim to equip graduates with the skills needed for success in the therapeutic field.

Our goal is to help students work effectively with people in crisis. The authors are both therapists and college professors and, therefore, see firsthand the importance of training and understanding trauma's effects. Our work with clients shows us the importance of underpinning theories and information combined with actual cases. Clinical practice sometimes poses questions that textbooks cannot answer, and academic preparation does not sufficiently introduce complex cases. Sometimes, a person is struggling with multiple issues and has several diagnosable conditions, and a neat, organized model does not fit the client's needs. Adaptability, flexibility, and reflexive thought become as crucial as our lectures. Novices entering the field discover what they do know but realize how little they know about helping people who are wounded.

In reflecting on current graduate education, we ask several questions. What is the emphasis? How do we know when our students are competent if we only query their intellectual knowledge without modeling excellent counseling skills? How do we build practice development, and when do we witness their growth? What lessons do they learn when they leave the academic world? Listening to licensed professional counselors about their development provides ideas on how to improve instruction for those entering the profession. These questions lead us to reconsider what we teach and how we do so. Is there a better way?

These future providers must learn to navigate an ever-changing world, and we know it is time to be genuine. Getting real means asking questions like "What is good enough?," "What makes one a competent therapist?," and "How can I affect the world around me?" Our classes grapple with these existential questions, novel ideas, and challenges in applying strategies. This process is vital in working with emerging professionals to learn how to help those who have experienced trauma. Getting genuine with clients means the new therapist will recognize when someone is authentic and fully present and learn that everything they do serves as an intervention. Our students observe professionals, how they act, dress, communicate, and arrange their offices, and those become part of treatment. They notice the interventions master therapists choose, how and when they are used, and why clinicians choose those tools.

In our andragogy, we envision students using their practical life lessons and excellent material. While knowing and memorizing the vast facts that inform counseling, we want to lead students in a richer discovery of the lessons needed through analysis and creativity. Adult students learn best using previous experience, current knowledge, and practical skills. As they sharpen their minds, they learn how their worldview influences their therapeutic encounters. Students strengthen their self-efficacy by unveiling what exists within themselves and exploring new ways of being. We stress the importance of knowing and understanding one's values. When a professional helper can self-reflect and resonate with their values, we believe this links to better decision-making and a more balanced approach to helping those who suffer. Emerging professionals will ask, "Can it be as simple as a connection?" Therapeutic alliance and connection are meaningful as clinicians extend care to people suffering from trauma, therefore making it more likely that the patient will receive appropriate and effective care.

Compassionate people come to this profession to offer hope and healing. However, without the proper trauma-informed training, they find themselves as the ones who are hurting. As our students, novice clinicians, and other professionals see a person struggling to find the words for the indescribable, they may become overwhelmed or dysregulated. It is difficult to explain the amount of discomfort these new professionals will ultimately face in their practices. It becomes challenging to maintain a healthy detachment sitting in the therapy chair. It is during those moments that therapists doubt their abilities. They wonder if they have entered the wrong profession or struggle to identify ways to aid the brokenhearted person who sits in their office. This doubt causes the sense of being an imposter. However, the novice can move from this position if fully prepared and trained.

These lessons in teaching graduates bring us to a place of humility and confrontation. Who else will do this work if we do not prepare them well? Therefore, we write this piece. This book does not aim to cover everything related to trauma comprehensively. It does not offer the satisfaction one would get from a five-course meal. Instead, it serves as the appetizer to stimulate curiosity for further knowledge. The text seeks to create a desire in others for more information, further training, and a greater appreciation of the importance of becoming trauma-informed. Other experts have come along who have deeper comprehension and more wisdom than we bring. Nevertheless, we, the ones sitting in a class of students who want to make a difference in this world but are anxious about how to do so, provide this text.

This book is created for seekers, those lacking education in trauma, and those who desire a brief overview. Use it as an interested person, student, educator, or researcher as a springboard to further exploration of traumatology. We hope the text offers what you need as an emerging professional in your field of work.

Acknowledgments

Trauma work is hard, and writing a book about trauma work is also hard. In the preface, we referenced getting real as trauma workers. This work is important and indispensable in our communities.

We are grateful to those who offered their review and feedback. We thank our associate vice president of academic affairs, Mary Millikin, for her trust and continuous encouragement and our department chair, Brian Andrews, for his unwavering support of this adventure.

This book is written with new counselors in mind. As such, we invited feedback from our current students and recent graduates. We are thankful to the following students and graduates for the extra time they gave in providing their reflections: Trixi Asher, Heather Clark, Rachel Dick, Samara Hamby, Tayah Holmes, Arissa Miller, and Shannon Smith. Chris Harrison and Mariah Nadeau, thank you for doing the tedious work for us. Our graduate students at Rogers State University in Claremore, Oklahoma give us inspiration and hope for the future as they become equipped and prepared to face a world full of possibilities.

Indebted, Michelle thanks Kathy, her trusted advisor and teaching partner. Together, they strive always to be good. Notable things she admires about Kathy are her zest for life, as she has energy in spades, and her unmatched kindness. Kathy is an inspirational, caring educator. Michelle is forever appreciative of her home team of Shawn, Grace, and Jack, who make all things possible and so incredibly worthwhile.

Kathy wishes to thank Michelle for her positivity and belief in a project that took time, energy, and unwavering commitment. Michelle Taylor's visionary leadership and belief in student growth are inspiring. Kathy also appreciates her spouse, who listens and offers feedback and lessons from his work as a chaplain and educator.

We thank our mentors, peers, and supervisors for what they taught us. Most importantly, we thank our clients throughout 60 years of clinical work, totaling more than 25,000 or more of them, for the lessons they taught us about providing the care they needed. We are tremendously appreciative of our publisher, Anna Moore, for her support of our effort and her commitment to this project.

Chapter One
Helping People with Trauma Experiences

Overview

Chapter 1: Helping People with Trauma Experiences explores the intricate nature of trauma, emphasizing the need for a comprehensive understanding and sensitivity among professionals who engage with individuals affected by trauma. The chapter outlines the prevalence of trauma, its diverse effects on individuals, and the significance of trauma-informed care and practice. It further explores the complex nature of defining trauma, addressing subjective and objective perspectives, and the challenges in categorizing trauma types. Chapter 1 notes the impact of trauma on individuals, various symptoms, and behavioral observations. It also presents the importance of salutogenesis in trauma work, accentuating the need to honor individual strengths and resources. In the section, A Flourishing Focus, the chapter introduces the salutogenesis model, highlighting a strength-based approach that focuses on resiliency and posttraumatic growth. In summary, the chapter provides a comprehensive overview of trauma, covering its multifaceted nature, impact, and the importance of trauma-informed care, and emphasizes resilience, underscoring the need for a strength-based approach in trauma work.

Trauma is Everywhere

No matter where you go, someone with a trauma history will cross your path. Even if the person you encounter does not meet the criteria for a trauma disorder, they may have a family member or close friend who has experienced extreme distress. When you observe someone acting negatively, you have a moment to determine how you will interpret their actions. Without a trauma perspective, it becomes easy to misjudge and

DOI: 10.4324/9781003463009-1

blame the person for their lack of responsibility, defective characteristics, or even their personality. Doing that may deprive you of a unique opportunity to bring hope and healing to a suffering person. Recall a previous visit to a public place. What observations did you make of people? Recently, we drove through a fast-food restaurant, where we ordered food and moved to the pickup window. The host did not look at us but handed us the bag, saying, "Here." Prior to being informed about trauma, we may have thought, "How rude. Someone needs to teach this person customer service skills." Now, we balance that with a caring perspective. They may require additional training, or they might be responding out of fear due to past traumatic experiences. Maybe they fought at home, cannot pay their bills, or have issues with pain or physical stamina. With trauma education, we see things differently and treat others more compassionately.

We are now aware that when we are missing essential information, our offers to help are misguided. In practicing self-reflection or self-supervision, we ask, "Whose need does this meet?" This question makes us examine whether our desire to help serves the other person we are concerned with or meets our need to be helpers. Can we refrain from helping if someone refuses, or will we take offense? How we treat people and what we think of them when they show up late for appointments or frequently cancel reveals our trauma sensitivity. Sometimes, our clients or colleagues remind us of how a narrow perspective of behavior is unhelpful and may damage those with trauma. We should acknowledge what we know but recognize the limits of our knowledge.

As we review the learning process, the steps we need to change to a trauma perspective include increasing trauma sensitivity, becoming trauma-informed, adopting a trauma-informed approach, and using evidence-based practices to help those with trauma. This requires learning about these terms and their differences in meaning before we are ready to provide care. However, confusion soon develops as one hears the myriads of terms used in traumatology. What is the distinction between trauma-sensitive and trauma-informed? These questions underscore the need for defining trauma.

What is Trauma?

In counseling classes, one of the most exciting subjects is trauma. We discuss questions: "What is trauma?" "Is trauma avoidable?" "Can anyone escape the reality of trauma?" Scull (2022) suggests that all humans will eventually experience a traumatic event. An example of the inevitability of trauma occurred with the coronavirus disease in 2019 (COVID-19). The world continues to experience different levels of trauma and loss from this pandemic, as evidenced by psychological shifts in crowded spaces and reactions to coughing. COVID-19 has challenged the world's view of trauma, primarily due to the global impact and implications wrought by this pandemic. The advent of COVID-19 introduced a new trauma type (Horesh & Brown, 2020; Kira et al., 2023). The world has collectively experienced trauma due to this event. Even without the pandemic, trauma is prevalent. In a study by the World Health Organization, approximately 70% of the global population has experienced one or more traumas (Kessler et al., 2017). Another study estimated that over 94 million U.S. adults have at least one exposure or more to a traumatic event (Forman-Hoffman et al., 2019). These statistics suggest that future clinicians and other professionals will need a comprehensive understanding of trauma to meet client or patient needs adequately.

Trauma comes from a Greek word meaning wound (Kolaitis & Olff, 2017). What does it mean for a person to have a wound? Does the size or degree of pain matter? Is it possible to have a cut and it not be a wound? This is what complicates trauma. How big does the trauma wound need to be? There is confusion about what constitutes trauma, which possibly leads people to believe their experience is less harmful than someone else's incident. Must a life-threatening event happen to be classified as trauma, or can intense situations traumatize? For instance, non-life-threatening automobile accidents can evoke traumatic symptoms in people. People describe family disruption or relocation as traumatic (Hanson & Lang, 2016). Who decides how trauma is defined? Even the terms referring to trauma care need clarification. What is the difference between trauma-informed care, practice, approaches, or sensitivity? These references communicate similar concepts yet differ from one another (Champine et al., 2019; Hanson & Lang, 2016). Students pursuing degrees in counseling frequently ask why there are so many differences in the definition of trauma. "Why cannot helping professionals come to an agreement on a common definition of trauma?" they inquire. In the most basic terms, future practitioners should remember that humans are complex beings who perceive experiences differently, adapting and evolving in various ways.

There are multiple reasons why trauma is challenging to define. How trauma is defined is dependent on socio-cultural, group, and individual perspectives. To understand what constitutes trauma may be related to cultural differences. Group influences, particularly political or social worldviews, will impact how we see trauma. Finally, people have unique experiences related to trauma. Some people may experience the same crisis, disaster, or difficult circumstance but may or may not view it as traumatic.

Trauma is Everywhere

Everyone has different appraisals of traumatic events. How can this be? In a podcast, food writer Ruth Reichl remarked that she does not know what others taste when they eat certain foods. In the interview, Reichl discusses that food experiences are easier to describe than flavor due to individual taste sensations. When Reichl writes, she attempts to transcend flavor so that her audience can understand the intangible nature of the sensory experience (Louis-Dreyfus, 2023). We use this reference in trauma teaching to show that individual perceptions of experiences vary greatly. Trauma can be explained in this way since trauma feels different to everyone, and those experiences may be disparate in severity and outlook. It is essential to understand that trauma is both tangible and intangible. Tangible losses may include physical injury, the loss of a person, and outcomes that cause harm, or visible injuries or scars on the person. Trauma can also include intangible elements, which are more abstract in that they cannot be touched physically, such as our private thoughts, feelings, and spiritual or sacred emotions. Knowing the concrete and subtle elements helps define trauma in subjective and objective ways.

Subjective Definitions

Future mental health practitioners are often eager to help clients recover from traumatic experiences. Some skilled experts or clinicians have faced traumatic events. Some enter the field because of their history of trauma. However, assumptions about trauma, how we define it, and how we treat it fluctuate among providers. Some think of trauma as a specific diagnosis, such as posttraumatic stress disorder (PTSD). In 2013, the American Psychiatric Association's version of the *Diagnostic and Statistical Manual for Mental Disorders* (*DSM*) expanded the criteria for PTSD, including not only actual or direct exposure to a potentially life-threatening situation but also the witnessing of such events. However, this poses difficulties for some whose experience does not fit such a definition. Robinson et al. (2023) define trauma as an extraordinary taxing event that undermines a person's sense of safety, while Starcevic (2019) describes trauma as an emotional reaction to a highly stressful situation.

One might face an overwhelming change, such as unemployment or divorce, which is not life-threatening. These may be stressful, and the individual may identify these circumstances as traumatic. In other cases, a person may be exposed to a life-threatening occurrence but never develop a complete set of symptoms as described in the *DSM-5-TR* (American Psychiatric Association, 2022). The symptoms may be sub-threshold PTSD and may interfere with life functioning. For example, military personnel tend to be under-diagnosed when their symptoms do not meet the full criteria for PTSD. Other individuals develop temporary stress symptoms from a traumatic event that quickly resolves. Some may have PTSD or experience traumatic events but do not report their trauma history to care providers (Morgan-López et al., 2023). Other people display many intense symptoms from traumatic events, leading to more severe pathology that requires intervention (SAMHSA, 2014). Some people are traumatized by an event, while others are not (Quiñones et al., 2022).

We believe in honoring a client's perspective of trauma. If the client believes they have suffered trauma, then we treat that as such. It is crucial to remember that practitioners are not investigators of whether a trauma occurred. Instead, providers focus on individual perceptions strongly associated with mental health outcomes (Rubin et al., 2014). How a person views the event and assigns meaning is essential in recovery. Future practitioners can accept the client's perception of such events without requiring accuracy or proof of that trauma. We acknowledge that some people recover quickly from traumatic experiences while others have lasting issues or symptoms. However, not all agree with this viewpoint, which relies on subjective components. Others argue that subjective experiences are inadequate in defining trauma and require objective measures (Boals, 2018). Practitioners, physicians, social workers, and first responders define, treat, and understand trauma differently. This disparity is apparent in the controversy in defining trauma.

Nurture Understanding

An expectant mother shared her story. On a sunny day in December 1985, two women in a local hospital had babies. It should have been a joyful occasion; unfortunately, it was not. The first woman, Sarah, had a baby boy who was quite ill. The doctor informed her that the baby had meningitis and would need hospitalization for several weeks. However, once treated, the baby could come home. Within 24 hours, the neonatologist updated the baby's prognosis. The specialist visited with Sarah and her husband, Dan. Their baby had hypoplastic left heart syndrome. The only possible solution was a series of operations offered by one hospital that was 1,600 miles away. The problem would be keeping the baby alive long enough and healing the meningitis so the baby could be a surgery candidate. The situation was grim since the life expectancy was one day to one month. There was not enough time, and the baby died on the fourth day. Sarah and Dan grieved for the loss of this baby, born full-term at 9 lbs., 6 oz.

The hospital staff had further sad news to deliver to another couple, April and Chris. Born at full term, their baby arrived with the umbilical cord wrapped around his neck. This baby did not survive. Two hopeful moms lost their babies during the same week. Two months later, a social worker connected the two women, thinking they could support one another since they had experienced similar traumatic events. Sarah and April met, but their perceptions were quite different. April cried, "Isn't this the most horrific thing that's ever happened?" Sarah hesitated and replied, "Yes, but I am okay because I felt prepared for it."

Sarah described how she felt forewarned intuitively before her baby's arrival. During her pregnancy, she prepared herself mentally and spiritually for the baby's due date, sensing that something was wrong. Sarah hoped that would not be the case, but with the preparation and support of her spouse, her acceptance of the tragedy helped her through the difficult time. Sarah also ascribed meaning to this tragedy as she reflected on the purpose it might serve for others as they witnessed how she and Dan responded to such a terrible event. April had no such preparation and little support from her spouse. The two women never met again, but through the years, Sarah often thought of April, wishing her peace. One might surmise that losing a child is the same experience for two mothers. However, this story shows that similar traumas have divergent effects.

- What contributes to a different view of a similar situation?
- Why do you believe Sarah and April's responses to fetal demise were so different?

Objective Definitions

The effort to operationalize trauma includes factors that delineate the intensity, significance, acuity of onset, duration, recurrence, and relationship to pre-trauma or premorbid conditions and individual characteristics (Spytska, 2023). The American Psychiatric Association (APA, 2022) defines PTSD as psychological distress that occurs upon direct or indirect exposure, witness of, or learning of a traumatic or stressful event to oneself, family member, or close friend wherein actual or threatened death is apparent. The problem with this definition is the lack of clarity on what constitutes a threat or an aversive experience (Dalenberg et al., 2017). This diagnosis is present in the category of Trauma- and Stressor-Related Disorders which also include Reactive Attachment Disorder, Disinhibited Social Engagement Disorder, Acute Stress Disorder, Adjustment Disorders, and Prolonged Grief Disorder. Each trauma- or stressor-related condition has individual criteria assigned to determine the diagnosis. These diagnoses have a close relationship due to extreme stressors (APA, 2022).

The Substance Abuse and Mental Health Services Administration (SAMHSA, 2014) views trauma as harmful, either emotionally or physically, resulting from a single event or series of events. Furthermore, these occurrences negatively impact an individual's functioning and well-being in many areas, including life's physical, emotional, mental, social, and spiritual aspects. SAMHSA (2014) distinguishes trauma by events, experiences, and effects. An event or events that involve severe neglect, physical or psychological abuse that is real or threatening, can happen once, more than once, or over time, are what cause trauma. An individual's experiences define the scope, intensity, and perspective of the traumatic incident. Ultimately, the negative consequences of the situation or situations could be long-lasting, including the breakdown of fundamental trust, alterations to cognitive functions, challenges in interpersonal and intrapersonal relationships, and modifications to the structure of the brain and physiological sequences (Compton & Schoeneberg, 2020). Experience determines whether it is a traumatic event. How trauma affects an individual depends on many factors. Effects can be long-lasting, and adverse outcomes can be immediate or delayed. The functional impact will determine how trauma is different for individuals. While diverse cultures define trauma in various ways, biologically, all humans experience stress similarly as the human body reacts with affect dysregulation and changes in structural functioning (Granieri et al., 2018). Moreover, trauma, in a universal sense, is an intense and unwanted experience.

Whether one works for or manages an organization that provides individual or familial care, being trauma-informed and providing trauma-informed practice is in the best interest of all people. There may be numerous factors that contribute to trauma, such as cultural and social variables, civil conflict, socioeconomic status, educational opportunities, and characteristics such as ethnicity, veteran status, and geographic origin (Forman-Hoffman et al., 2019). One person's perception of the same traumatic event can be accepted and processed. For another, it can be debilitating, leaving a client unable to move forward with everyday routines. To align how a client processes different traumatic events and create an effective treatment plan, future practitioners

Trauma is Everywhere

must be able to differentiate between different types of traumas as we seek deeper understanding.

Cultivate Knowledge

After reading about the difficulty in defining trauma, try creating your own definition.

- Try to write your definition in two or three sentences.
- If you had a client who had a traumatic experience, how would you explain trauma to them?

Trauma Perspectives

Trauma can have lifelong effects on specific individuals. When a person has a traumatic experience, it impacts their view of themselves, others, and the world around them. They may have difficulties with feeling safe despite being sheltered at the moment. They may mistrust others, especially healthcare providers, and any slight breach of trust confirms that implicit suspicion (Bell et al., 2019). Living in a world that feels uncontrollable, trauma survivors grasp power and control, and relationships become complicated as they may misinterpret the actions or words of others (SAMHSA, 2014). The world becomes a place of fear for some people and understanding that guides you in knowing that what you offer must be done with precision, focus, intention, and commitment.

A trauma perspective begins with this awareness and continues to develop with self-reflection and knowledge of the people who have not received adequate care, particularly those marginalized populations who do not have access to the best treatment modalities and continue to live in a traumatized culture (Brissett et al., 2023; Gherardi et al., 2020; Isobel, 2023). Being a trauma-sensitive professional means recognizing the deleterious effects of trauma and seeing the possibility of growth. Once we become trauma-sensitive, we can learn about trauma-informed care.

Moving to a broader structure of understanding trauma means becoming informed on how to develop organizations that use a trauma-informed framework and provide trauma-informed care. With the realization of the widespread impact of trauma, systems recognize trauma symptoms in people, can respond in integrative ways to help others and make intentional efforts to avoid re-traumatization (Champine et al., 2022;

Harris & Fallot, 2001). Trauma-informed care means developing policies, programs, and practices that inform services and care delivery system-wide in organizations (Hanson & Lang, 2016). This understanding requires reframing everyone's view (Champine et al., 2022). Trauma-informed care requires sensitivity to patients, providers, and staff and relies on six basic principles: safety, choice, collaboration, empowerment, trustworthiness, and consideration of cultural, historical, and gender issues (SAMHSA, 2014). A trauma-informed agency views problems within the context of a client's past traumatic experiences (Knight, 2019; Levenson, 2020). Staff knowledge, sensitivity, and patient satisfaction increase when organizations provide trauma-informed training. Other positive outcomes of this training include increased trauma screening, increased patient perception of decision-making, increased patient satisfaction, and reduced seclusions, restraints, and assaults on staff (Purtle, 2018). Some practitioners believe that a trauma-informed approach does not sufficiently address concerns related to embarrassment and indignity and thus recommend training staff to be sensitive to issues of shame and guilt (Dolezal & Gibson, 2022).

Those who are trauma-informed can implement trauma-informed practices in clinical work and become skilled at integrating the role trauma has played in the lives of others (SAMHSA, 2014). In essence, it becomes easier to go from trauma-informed care to trauma-informed interventions that elicit positive progress in healing. This orientation allows for holistic treatment of people at systemic levels, training staff to understand that trauma stress affects the brain and body. It also helps organizations realize that their employees may have a trauma history, and creating a safe space empowers and protects them. This perspective focuses on understanding a person's experiences rather than identifying faults, seeing symptoms as adaptive strategies, and providing collaborative services (Kimberg & Wheeler, 2019). When helpers view things from this lens, they point to hope and restoration (Figure 1.1).

Trauma-informed care is an organizational effort, while trauma-informed practice is more accurately descriptive of how a clinician understands trauma, the trauma diagnoses, and symptoms (Szczygiel, 2018). It includes clinical assessment, diagnosis, and interventions for patients with trauma (Levenson, 2020). In trauma-focused practice, providers center on addressing the trauma experience with clients (Knight, 2019). Trauma-specific services or trauma-informed practices become the type of interventions used to address trauma symptoms. This level of care seeks to offer the best evidence-based interventions and approaches for trauma treatment (Brissett et al., 2023; DeCandia & Guarino, 2015; SAMHSA, 2014). This foundation sets the stage for

Trauma Perspectives

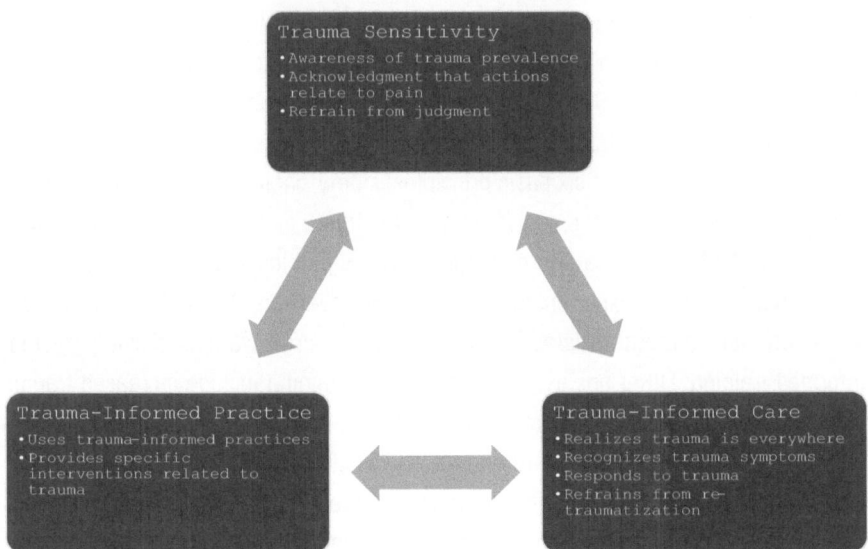

FIGURE 1.1   Trauma Perspectives.

(Champine et al., 2022; Harris & Fallot, 2001; SAMHSA, 2014).

any professional who provides care to those with traumatic experiences. While understanding the various ways to define trauma and the assorted perspectives, classification of trauma types is needed.

Trauma Types

Delineating trauma types is dependent on taxonomy or ways in which helpers or professionals classify trauma. Some scholars provide types of traumas based on a categorical framework of the event or source occurrence, criterion-based descriptors, symptoms, or development-based trauma. An official taxonomy for trauma acceptable to all helping professions is yet undetermined (Levin-Aspenson & Greene, 2024). Trauma types can be unwieldy due to exploring or explaining multiple views. However, a general idea of how to order trauma may help determine ways to assess, treat, research, and develop policies of prevention and intervention.

One way to clarify trauma is by event type or its source. There are several categories: adverse childhood experiences, natural disasters, human-created or human-caused disasters, historical trauma, and mass violence. Adverse childhood experiences (ACEs) are potential traumatic events that occur during childhood. These include child maltreatment, such as physical, emotional, or sexual abuse; physical or emotional neglect; and household dysfunction, such as divorce, substance abuse, interpersonal violence, incarcerated relative, or a family member with a mental illness. Additional ACEs include bullying, community violence, neighborhood safety, racism, and living in foster care (Cronholm et al., 2015; Tomlinson et al., 2024).

When viewing trauma as a stress reaction to a threatening event, adults describe different traumas that have occurred during their lifetime. These include natural events, such as accidents, technological catastrophes, and intentional acts. Natural or disaster traumas include tornados, lightning strikes, wildfires, earthquakes, hurricanes, typhoons, blizzards, floods, tsunamis, physical illness, or an epidemic, such as the worldwide COVID-19 pandemic. Such events affect large population samples (SAMHSA, 2014). Human-created or human-caused disasters include accidents and technological catastrophes such as structural collapses, airplane crashes, mine collapses, gas explosions, electrocution, machine-related accidents, oil spills, and sports-related deaths. Intentional acts include terrorism, sexual assault, homicide or suicide, human trafficking, torture, home invasion or robbery, and genocide. These are acts imposed on a human by another human being or group of humans (Hathaway et al., 2010). Historical trauma, or intergenerational trauma, refers to the traumatic experiences of historically marginalized people, such as African Americans, Native Americans, and Asian Americans (Nagata et al., 2024). Mass violence includes situations in which large numbers of people are wounded or killed, such as school shootings, warfare, or political unrest.

The *Diagnostic and Statistical Manual of Mental Health Disorders 5th Edition Text Revision* (*DSM-5-TR*; APA, 2022) describes trauma as it affects a person's psychological self. However, this viewpoint ignores existential threats to a person's sense of identity, vital for human growth and development. This categorization is helpful when requiring clear criteria to diagnose an individual with a mental health disorder but neglects the basic needs of individuals for meaning and purpose (Kira, 2022). Many professions refer to trauma as acute, chronic, or complex. Acute trauma may occur from a single incident, whereas chronic trauma appears when the trauma is repeated or prolonged, such as with domestic violence or abuse. Complex trauma refers to exposure to multiple traumatic events occurring over a prolonged period (Feriante & Sharma, 2023). Terr (1991) suggests two types of traumas: Type 1 and Type 2. Type 1 trauma is single-event trauma, whereas Type 2 trauma refers to an ongoing event or multiple traumatic situations (Compton & Schoeneberg, 2020).

Trauma Perspectives

An innovative way to categorize trauma is through the development-based trauma framework. This perspective views trauma as an event or series of conditions that present an existential threat to a person and their identity. This taxonomy includes five groups of traumas: achievement trauma, identity trauma, interdependence trauma, attachment trauma, and survival trauma. There are subtypes within each category (Kira, 2021). Achievement trauma occurs when an individual fails to meet a personal goal essential to social survival, such as being laid off from work or prolonged unemployment, a substantial loss of money, valuables, or health, or substantial failure to achieve life goals. Identity trauma is a sense of helplessness that arises when an individual exists in circumstances where there is no foreseeable or immediate escape. This type of trauma depletes an individual's independence and deflates their sense of personal identity. Examples of this type include sexual and physical abuse, domestic violence, rape, slavery, being a prisoner of war, undergoing torture, or genocide.

A third type of trauma threatens the connections or social network of an individual, particularly those that provide emotional and social support or meaning in life. Examples of interdependence trauma include changing schools frequently, moving locales frequently, and the refugee experience (Kira, 2021). Attachment trauma occurs with a break in the bond between child and primary caregiver. This trauma type may be due to abuse, neglect, lack of affection, or responsiveness to the child from the caregiver. Finally, survival trauma is due to an event that poses a direct or indirect threat to oneself or significant others. This type could include witnessing or participating in war, attempted suicide, homicide, vehicle accident, violent crimes, or natural or manufactured disasters (Kira, 2021). How trauma is typed is an area where further consideration and research could benefit those who endure significant events. Differences in trauma symptoms depend on what occurred, how long it lasted, and the severity. Trauma taxonomy informs symptom occurrence, remission methods, and recovery attainment. Trauma exposure has both short-term and long-term consequences (SAMHSA, 2014) (Figure 1.2).

Trauma Effects

People have different responses to traumatic stress. Clients may seek help for wounds to the body, mind, or spirit. Symptoms may present through physiological changes, behavioral problems, emotional responses, cognitive distortions, disrupted relational

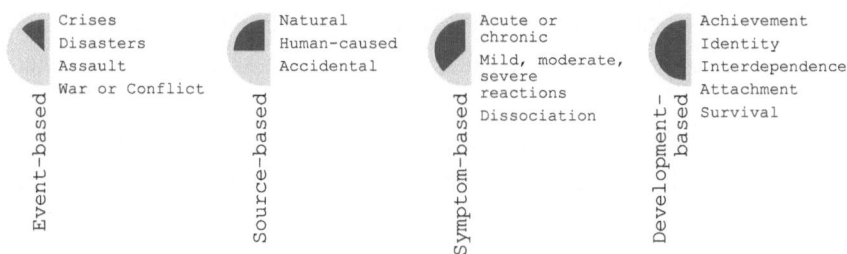

FIGURE 1.2   Trauma Typology.

(Kira, 2021).

connections, and daily functioning. Physiological changes may include hypervigilance, stomach problems, appetite disturbance, shakiness, headaches, or worsening health conditions. Sleep disruption may occur as some experience nightmares (APA, 2022). Clients describe physiological symptoms such as dry mouth, diarrhea, perspiration, trembling, heart palpitations, and problems in breathing (Holtzhausen, 2017).

Behavioral problems may occur as increased substance use, such as drinking more alcohol, using illicit drugs, misusing prescription medicine, or smoking more (Holtzhausen, 2017; Park et al., 2017; U.S. Department of Veterans Affairs National Center for PTSD, 2024). The U.S. Department of Veterans Affairs National Center for PTSD (VA, 2024) describes other behavioral changes such as avoidance or hypervigilance. Certain individuals are easily startled, reacting to the slightest sound, and constantly feeling vigilant. The emotional symptoms may include nervousness, sadness, shock, numbness, or detachment. Others may experience emotional distress when faced with reminders of the traumatic event or something that symbolizes the trauma (Holtzhausen, 2017; VA, 2024).

Cognitive symptoms may include intrusive thoughts or memories, flashbacks, and negative changes in thoughts (APA, 2022). Trauma can evoke negative changes in thinking, such as the inability to recall essential facets of the traumatic event or viewing oneself or the world negatively. Some clients experience exaggerated blame, guilt, or shame, while some are anxious, depressed, or suicidal (Park et al., 2017). Others feel a sense of disorientation and confusion. Cognitive symptoms may include viewing the world, people, or oneself differently or difficulty trusting others (Sweeton, 2019).

Mind and spirit references from clients are visible in the disconnection between self and others and expressing loss of purpose and meaning. Clients may also be isolated

Trauma Perspectives

and experience loneliness and abandonment (Holtzhausen, 2017; Park et al., 2017). People who experience traumatic stress may have increasing difficulty in relationships with family or co-workers. Traumatic stress reactions appear in marital problems, which the helper may view as a communication problem or as family dysfunction, either as enmeshment or disengagement, unaware that traumatic stress reactions are the reason. Others may have difficulty functioning at home or work (VA, 2024). People who endure complex trauma may struggle with trust, social safety, power and control, self-esteem, and relationships (Isobel, 2023; VA, 2024).

Trauma disrupts a person on many levels and in different ways. How people experience it and what symptoms develop may vary based on the type of trauma. How different traumas affect people is currently being explored. Survival trauma tends to affect memory and inhibition directly, whereas attachment trauma affects working memory but not inhibition (Kira et al., 2022). Those who experience prolonged or complex trauma tend to have more dissociative experiences (Granieri et al., 2018). The International Society for the Study of Trauma and Dissociation (ISSTD, 2023) states that many describe dissociation as if something overtakes them. They might sense something happening yet feel like spectators in a movie, like depersonalization. This altered state of consciousness may include a sense of derealization as if one were not present. Some individuals suffer from temporary amnesia, with no recollection of events during that period. This dissociation affects memory, identity, and perception (ISSTD, 2023). Other differences in what symptoms develop may be related to family environment or sociological factors, such as having a parent with a substance use problem or psychiatric issue, poverty, or frequent moves or changes (Schimmenti, 2017). When a person experiences trauma, their symptoms may be misinterpreted as the behaviors are ascribed to personality characteristics (Munjiza et al., 2019) (Table 1.1).

What is impressive is how many people exhibit positive psychological changes as a result. Tedeschi and Calhoun (1995) describe this as posttraumatic growth. This parallel process leads to increased self-awareness and confidence, openness toward others, and a paradigm change that opens new possibilities (Tedeschi et al., 2018). In practice, clients who experience trauma are adaptive and resilient. In all trauma training, we must honor the client's courage, bravery, and resilience at the beginning of trauma work while we learn how to offer beneficial and effective care.

TABLE 1.1   Behavioral Observations of Trauma Reactions

A person who has experienced trauma may:	This may be due to:
Seem disrespectful	Poor social skills, inability to connect, distractibility
Misunderstand or refuse to follow instructions; ask for repetition of instructions or avoid asking for instruction	Reduced concentration skills, poor memory, reduced cognitive skills, fear, lack of trust
Avoid eye contact, appointments, not return phone calls	Avoidance of things, places, memories, or inquiries about their trauma
Be easily startled, nervous, twitch, shake	Overactivation of the sympathetic nervous system; hypervigilance; fear
Act as if they do not care or do not trust or seem paranoid, argue	Poor social skills, inability to connect, inability to trust
Withhold information, look away, avoid eye contact	Shame, disappointment, fear; poor memory
Arrive late	Sleep disturbance, nightmares, panic attacks
Use substances	Self-medication of symptoms
Make hasty decisions that are not in their best interest	Increased impulsiveness due to impaired cognitive abilities
Be unable to remember situations accurately, or change their story frequently	Decreased memories; flashbacks; high distractibility
Be reluctant to participate	Fear or anxiety
Defend the perpetrator, refuse to cooperate, ask for the case to be dismissed	Impaired social abilities

Source: Albrink (2023) and Sweeton (2019).

Tending Your Technique

How do we put it together? Answer the following questions:

How can you discern the difference between a rude person and one with a history of trauma?

Which symptoms do you think are the most problematic?

How do these symptoms determine the course of treatment?

A Flourishing Focus

When we study how humans develop, we learn that growth is a continuous process. We do not arrive fully equipped to navigate life. Instead, life brings questions, trials, and tests to encourage the full expansion of our potential. People become creative, resourceful, and whole through their experiences, choices, and learning. This development requires disequilibrium, or repeated births and deaths of preconceptions, or, as Jung described it, "enantiodromia" (1959, p. 252). This is the unconscious work of opposites, the dialectic of creation and destruction, building up and tearing down, learning trust and mistrust, being intrapersonal and interpersonal, engaging in life and detaching for protection.

Comparing this to plant life, we see how this occurs. The seed arrives dormant but ready to germinate. The possibility for a flourishing plant is present but is influenced by environmental factors that are far more complex than one realizes. It is not just a matter of water, light, and soil. Instead, the water content, light condition, surrounding temperature, and soil composition are vital (Yang et al., 2020). While all plants need similar elements, each need varying compositions of those elements. However, the process of germination begins once the planted seed breaks open and a shoot emerges. The seed must experience disequilibrium, or a change in its current state. This is when transformation occurs.

Trauma causes disequilibrium. The experience of trauma may be catastrophic for some, but for others, the tragedy results in posttraumatic growth, or a flourishing effect. Encouraging a salutogenic approach to clients may involve asking, "How did your world change?" and "What gave you the courage to survive?" after asking about what happened. In this approach, the provider or helper honors the individual's strengths and resources (Ginwright, 2018). The salutogenic model, introduced by Antonovsky (1987), proposes that all experiences in life shape one's sense of coherence or essential view of survival. This perspective encompasses three facets: life is comprehensible, manageable, and meaningful. This understanding aids people or eases distress when facing seemingly insurmountable events (Mittelmark & Bauer, 2022). Frankl (1946) describes this sense of coherence in *Man's Search for Meaning*, written while imprisoned at Auschwitz during World War II. This broader view of events enables traumatized individuals to make sense of their experiences and informs how they might view past and future events (King & Hicks, 2021).

History is replete with people and nations that thrive after traumatic events. It is not the occurrence that produces resilience but rather the struggle to learn how to manage these critical incidents (Henson et al., 2021). The challenge for traumatized individuals and populations is their reconsideration of how the world operates and how their former beliefs are limiting (Calhoun & Tedeschi, 2013). Developing new lives may take months or even years, involving cognitive reappraisal. They first must question why the event happened and how the trauma impacted them. Along with this cognitive process is the search for meaning (Frankl, 1946). However, to actively process, individuals must use their available internal and external resources to support their exploration.

Trauma may be catastrophic for some, but for others, tragedy induces posttraumatic growth. In *Unraveling the Mysteries of Health: How People Manage Stress and Stay Well*, Antonovsky coined salutogenesis. Antonovsky's medical sociology background led him to seek patterns of behaviors and decisions that move a client toward health (Antonovsky, 1987). Historically, the medical training model focuses on pathogenesis or the development of disease (Burns, 2014). However, some consider this model a barrier to the healing process. Salutogenesis focuses on what creates wellness or healing (Burns, 2014; Mittelmark & Bauer, 2022). Antonovsky emphasized that people are not broken but are experts on themselves. In applying salutogenesis, the helper encourages the individual to move from a state of perceived brokenness to acceptance (Bauer et al., 2020). In the salutogenic model, practitioners focus on maintaining good health and positive ways to strive for well-being (Bhattacharya et al., 2020).

A salutogenic approach to clients may involve asking, "What is right with you?" after asking about what happened. In this approach, the provider or helper is honoring the strength of an individual or group (Ginwright, 2018). This healing model is a worldview that posits life is manageable when a person accesses available resources to cope with stressors (Mittelmark & Bauer, 2022). In other words, people have an enduring ability to see that the world is intelligible and significant (Huss & Samson, 2018). This view does not minimize the consequences of trauma, nor does it displace the responsibility of oppressive acts, but instead emphasizes a human's ability for growth. According to the sense of coherence, individuals develop generalized and specific resistance resources during childhood and adolescence that aid in coping with stressors. As people deal with stressful life events, this strength of coherence may weaken temporarily but strengthen as individuals successfully manage stress (Braun-Lewensohn et al., 2013). When facing adverse events, generalized resistance resources or adequate resources and coping skills serve a moderating effect on posttraumatic stress (Schäfer et al., 2019). Using a salutogenic approach decreases the severity of PTSD symptoms due to increased self-efficacy, resiliency, and meaning-making (Schäfer et al., 2019). When individuals have an increased sense of coherence, their PTSD symptoms become less intense (Schäfer et al., 2019). This discovery

A Flourishing Focus

means that providers may need to include this approach for successful recovery for their clients or patients. Future practitioners can assist clients with choices and decisions that can lead a person to improved health outcomes.

The focus on salutogenesis is vital to resilience. In this text, we call this *A Flourishing Focus* to demonstrate how powerful resilience, or posttraumatic growth, can be. This reminder points to the most potent tool that trauma workers and people who experience trauma possess. Resilience may differ for each but will reside in the positive outlook, the internal resources, external support, and the discovery of meaningful connections. Supporting a client or patient's current strengths and support system is beneficial and asking them to analyze the purpose of their experience is helpful.

Gather Self-Awareness

- Please describe what you learned about trauma in this chapter and how it affects you.
- What did you learn about yourself in reading this chapter?
- As you reflect on your traumatic events, how have they changed you?

Chapter Summary

Chapter 1 provided an overview of trauma, highlighting its prevalence and diverse effects on individuals. The chapter stressed the importance of professionals having a comprehensive understanding and sensitivity when working with traumatized individuals. It explored the challenges in defining and categorizing trauma types. It provided definitions of trauma in subjective and objective ways. Trauma perspectives such as trauma sensitivity, trauma-informed care, and trauma-informed practices were outlined as the chapter discussed trauma symptoms, behavior, and posttraumatic growth. Chapter 1 introduced the concept of salutogenesis, focusing on resilience and posttraumatic growth. It emphasized the importance of a strength-based approach in trauma work. The chapter included a list of resources related to trauma-informed care. In completing the activities, you responded to questions related to various cases of *Nurture Understanding*. In the activity *Cultivate Knowledge*, you defined trauma and how to explain it to clients. Through *Tending Your Techniques*, you had the opportunity to reflect on your behavioral observations and understanding of trauma symptoms, and in *Ripen Self-Awareness*, you reflected on the reading and how it impacts you.

How to Use This Book

The topics in this textbook include a discussion about trauma and its definition, the neurobiology of trauma and empathy, assessment and diagnosis, evidence-based treatments, managing suicide, crisis, and disaster, dealing with the inevitable challenges of the work, and bringing second-order change to the world around. The information provided to you arrives in nine chapters. *Chapter 1: Helping People with Trauma Experiences* explores the universality of trauma, the definition of trauma, the various perspectives of trauma, and the importance of resilience. In *Chapter 2: The Neurobiology of Trauma*, we discuss how trauma affects the body, how our understanding of this neurobiology developed, and the role of neurobiology in resilience. One of our favorite topics comes in *Chapter 3: Burnout, Secondary Traumatic Stress, and Empathy*, as we explore how therapists are at risk in working with traumatized individuals. We explain how this happens and offer wisdom and resources for prevention.

Moving to *Chapter 4: Assessment*, we offer advice on how to begin with assessment in trauma work and what tools provide help in this stage. *Chapter 5: Diagnosing Trauma* explores the history of trauma diagnosis, how posttraumatic stress disorder (PTSD) has changed throughout time, how acute stress disorder developed, and the controversy of complex PTSD. Finally, this chapter examines how trauma disorders are easily confused with other diagnoses. In *Chapter 6: Evidence-Based Treatments*, we offer guidelines and best practices for treating adults, children, adolescents, and military personnel. In this chapter, we briefly explain four primary treatment approaches, Cognitive Behavioral Therapy, Cognitive Processing Therapy, Prolonged Exposure Therapy, and Eye Movement and Desensitization Reprocessing (EMDR), as well as parent or caregiver modalities.

Chapter 7: Suicide, Crisis, and Disaster, offers research about these phenomena, including the prevalence, risk factors, and warning signs. This chapter discusses suicide assessment and intervention, along with the occurrence of non-suicidal self-injury. Interventions for crisis and disaster are offered, including an explanation of Psychological First Aid and Critical Incident Stress Management and Debriefing. In *Chapter 8: Challenges in Trauma Work*, we look at the various barriers that arise when we work with traumatized people, including challenges that occur at individual, clinician, organizational, and systemic levels. The book ends with *Chapter 9: Becoming Effective Providers in Resilient Communities*, wherein we address how to change paradigms in our society, what it means to be a trauma-informed society, how that applies to various professional roles, and how to become effective in trauma work.

Chapter Summary

The reader will notice that we stray from the strict application of American Psychological Association (APA) grammar and pronoun usage guidelines. While our citations and references are formatted accordingly, within the chapters, we write conversationally, just as if we are present in the room with a reader. This way, it captures your attention as a reader and engages you in interaction with the text. We invite you to read, question, or argue with the text as that dialogue enhances your learning. As such, we offer activities throughout each chapter to challenge your thinking. These activities are growth opportunities labeled *Nurture Understanding*, *Cultivate Knowledge*, *Tending Your Technique*, and *Ripen Self-Awareness*.

This text applies emerging and current scientific information that can be applied to everyday clinical situations for multiple healthcare professionals, from nursing to clinical mental health.

In the *Nurture Understanding* activities, we offer case studies and examples designed to help learners view scenarios and assemble knowledge of theory and practice with contextual insights dealing with client outcomes. In our case studies and interviews, composite cases are offered, fictional names are used, and details and information have been altered to protect the anonymity of those involved. The cases and interviews do not represent actual individuals and should not be construed as such.

We ask you to critically reflect on the reading material through the activities, *Cultivate Knowledge*. In this activity, we test your recall and ask you to analyze it. In doing so, you are building on the notions that trauma can be treated effectively and ensuring that you apprehend that trauma is particular and personal. When the text offers you *Tending Your Technique*, this encourages you to view trauma critically while applying what you have learned with counseling techniques to help you sharpen your skills in aiding others to change, grow, and achieve.

At the end of each chapter, we ask that readers *Ripen Self-Awareness* by utilizing reflective questions to coalesce content knowledge. These questions seek to build on the foundation of trauma-informed practices. As people, we all learn from our journeys, and we hope you will keep striving toward competency with compassion as you work with traumatized individuals.

You will notice throughout the textbook that we include a salutogenic framework. The application of salutogenesis, or what health becomes for those who experience trauma, focuses on resilience. We believe people are not broken vessels waiting to be glued back to normal but rather creative, resourceful, and whole individuals who can transcend damaging, ugly, and even evil circumstances. Through this emphasis, we offer encouragement and hope to all who experience the inevitability of traumatic events.

Chapter Review

Please respond to the following questions.

1. What is the importance of trauma-informed care and practice?
2. What challenges are involved in defining and categorizing trauma types?
3. What is salutogenesis, and how does it relate to trauma?
4. What resources are provided for trauma-informed care and education?

Key Term Assessment

Review the following terms and try to explain each concept.

- Trauma
- Trauma types
- Resilience
- Salutogenesis

Resources

The following resources may be helpful. At the time of this writing, they were accessible through the links provided.

- SAMHSA's Key Ingredients for Successful Trauma-Informed Care Implementation https://www.samhsa.gov/sites/default/files/programs_campaigns/childrens_mental_health/atc-whitepaper-040616.pdf
- SAMHSA offers this brief to guide organizations in best practices who desire to offer trauma-informed care. The brief uses interviews with national experts on trauma-informed care and creates a framework for organizational and clinical care that can be applied in a system that offers physical and mental health care to patients with a trauma history.
- SAMHSA's Concept of Trauma and Guidance for a Trauma-Informed Approach https://store.samhsa.gov/sites/default/files/d7/priv/sma14-4884.pdf

Chapter Summary

- SAMHSA provides this resource as a guide for organizations who desire to provide a trauma-informed approach. This 20-page document discusses the background of trauma, the concept and difficulty defining trauma, SAMHSA's concept of trauma, and the key assumptions and principles of a trauma-informed approach. Following this information, the document discusses guidance for implementing a trauma-informed approach in organizations and explores a trauma-informed perspective within the context of a community.

References

Albrink, L. G. (2023). Trauma-informed legal advocacy. *Wake Forest Journal of Law & Policy, 13*, 67–102. https://heinonline.org/HOL/P?h=hein.journals/wfjlapo13&i=80

American Psychiatric Association (APA). (2022). *Diagnostic and statistical manual of mental disorders: DSM-5-TR*. American Psychiatric Association.

Antonovsky, A. (1987). *Unraveling the mystery of health: How people manage stress and stay well*. Jossey-Bass Publishers.

Bauer, G. F., Roy, M., Bakibinga, P., Contu, P., Downe, S., Eriksson, M., Espnes, G. A., Jensen, B. B., Canal, D. J., Lindström, B., Mana, A., Mittelmark, M. B., Morgan, A. R., Pelikan, J. M., Saboga-Nunes, L., Sagy, S., Shorey, S., Vaandrager, L., & Vinje, H. F. (2020). Future directions for the concept of salutogenesis: A position article. *Health Promotion International, 35*(2), 187–195. https://doi.org/10.1093/heapro/daz057

Bell, V., Robinson, B., Katona, C., Fett, A. K., & Shergill, S. (2019). When trust is lost: The impact of interpersonal trauma on social interactions. *Psychological Medicine, 49*(6), 1041–1046. https://doi.org/10.1017/S0033291718001800

Bhattacharya, S., Pradhan, K. B., Bashar, M. A., Tripathi, S., Thiyagarajan, A., Srivastava, A., & Singh, A. (2020). Salutogenesis: A bona fide guide towards health preservation. *Journal of Family Medicine and Primary Care, 9*(1), 16–19. https://doi.org/10.4103/jfmpc.jfmpc_260_19

Boals, A. (2018). Trauma in the eye of the beholder: Objective and subjective definitions of trauma. *Journal of Psychotherapy Integration, 28*(1), 77–89. https://doi.org/10.1037.int0000050

Braun-Lewensohn, O., Sagy, S., Sabato, H., & Galili, R. (2013). Sense of coherence and sense of community as coping resources of religious adolescents before and after the disengagement from the Gaza Strip. *The Israel Annals of Psychiatry and Related Disciplines, 50*(2), 110–117.

Brissett, D. I., Davies, S. H., & Sit, L. (2023). Reimagining no-shows as a symptom and not a diagnosis: A strength-based, trauma-sensitive approach. *Pediatrics, 151*(6). https://doi.org/10.1542/peds.2022-057590

Burns, H. (2014). What causes wellness [YouTube video]. *Tedx Glasgow*. https://www.youtube.com/watch?v=yEh3JG74C6s

Calhoun, L. G., & Tedeschi, R. G. (2013). *Posttraumatic growth in clinical practice*. Routledge.

Champine, R. B., Hoffman, E. R., Matlin, S. L., Strambler, M. J., & Tebes, J. K. (2022). "What does it mean to be trauma-informed?": A mixed-methods study of a trauma-informed community initiative. *Journal of Child and Family Studies, 31*, 459–472. https://doi.org/10.1007/s10826-021-02195-9

Champine, R. B., Lang, J. M., Nelson, A. M., Hanson, R. F., & Tebes, J. K. (2019). Systems measures of a trauma-informed approach: A systematic review. *American Journal of Community Psychology, 64*(3–4), 418–437. https://doi.org/10.1002/ajcp.12388

Compton, L., & Schoeneberg, C. (2020). *Preparing for trauma work in clinical mental health.* Taylor & Francis.

Cronholm, P. F., Forke, C. M., Wade, R., Bair-Merritt, M. H., Davis, M., Harkins-Schwarz, M., Pachter, L. M., & Fein, J. A. (2015). Adverse childhood experiences: Expanding the concept of adversity. *American Journal of Preventive Medicine, 49*(3), 354–361. https://doi.org/10.1016/j.amepre.2015.02.001

Dalenberg, C. J., Straus, E., & Carlson, E. B. (2017). Defining trauma. In S. N. Gold (Ed.), *APA handbook of trauma psychology: Foundations in knowledge.* American Psychological Association.

DeCandia, C., & Guarino, K. (2015). Trauma-informed care: An ecological response. *Journal of Child and Youth Care Work, 25*, 7–32. https://doi.org/10.5195/jcycw.2015.69

Dolezal, L., & Gibson, M. (2022). Beyond a trauma-informed approach and towards a shame-sensitive practice. *Humanities & Social Sciences Communications, 9*, 214. https://doi.org/10.1057/s41599-022-01227-z

Feriante, J., & Sharma, N. P. (2023). *Acute and chronic mental health trauma.* StatPearls Publishing. https://www.ncbi.nlm.nih.gov/books/NBK594231/

Forman-Hoffman, V., Batts, K., Bose, J., Glasheen, C., Hirsch, E., Yu, F., & Hedden, S. (2019). Correlates of exposure to potentially traumatic experiences: Results from a national household survey. *Psychological Trauma: Theory, Research, Practice, and Policy, 11*(3), 360–367.

Frankl, V. E. (1946). *Man's search for meaning* (Trans. I. Lasch). Beacon Press.

Gherardi, S. A., Flinn, R. E., & Jaure, V. B. (2020). Trauma-sensitive schools and social justice: A critical analysis. *The Urban Review, 52*, 482–504. https://doi.org/10.1007/s11256-020-00553-3

Ginwright, S. (2018, May 31). The future of healing: Shifting from trauma-informed care to healing-centered engagement. *Medium.* https://ginwright.medium.com/the-future-of-healing-shifting-from-trauma-informed-care-to-healing-centered-engagement-634f557ce69c

Granieri, A., Guglielmucci, F., Costanzo, A., Caretti, V., & Schimmenti, A. (2018). Trauma-related dissociation is linked with maladaptive personality functioning. *Frontiers in Psychiatry, 9*, 206. https://doi.org/10.3389/fpsyt.2018.00206

References

Hanson, R. F., & Lang, J. (2016). A critical look at trauma-informed care among agencies and systems serving maltreated youth and their families. *Child Maltreatment, 21*(2), 95–100. https://doi.org/10.1177/1077559516635274

Harris, M., & Fallot, R. (Eds.). (2001). *New directions for mental health services: Using trauma theory to design service systems.* Jossey-Bass.

Hathaway, L. M., Boals, A., & Banks, J. B. (2010). PTSD symptoms and dominant emotional response to a traumatic event: An examination of *DSM-IV* criterion A2. *Anxiety, Stress, and Coping, 23,* 119–126. https://doi.org/10.1080/10615800902818771

Henson, C., Truchot, D., & Canevello, A. (2021). What promotes posttraumatic growth? A systematic review. *European Journal of Trauma & Dissociation, 5*(4). https://doi.org/10.1016/j.ejtd.2020.100195

Holtzhausen, L. (2017). Addiction – A brain disorder or a spiritual disorder. *Mental Health and Addiction Research, 2*(1), 1–7. https://doi.org/10.15761/MHAR.1000128

Horesh, D., & Brown, A. D. (2020). Traumatic stress in the age of COVID-19: A call to close critical gaps and adapt to new realities. *Psychological Trauma: Theory, Research, Practice, and Policy, 12*(4), 331–335. https://doi.org/10.1037/tra0000592

Huss, E., & Samson, T. (2018). Drawing on the arts to enhance salutogenic coping with health-related stress and loss. *Frontiers in Psychology, 9,* Article 1612. https://doi.org/10.3389/fpsyg.2018.01612

International Society for the Study of Trauma and Dissociation (ISSTD). (2023). *Dissociation FAQs.* https://www.isst-d.org/resources/dissociation-faqs/

Isobel, S. (2023). Trauma and the perinatal period: A review of the theory and practice of trauma-sensitive interactions for nurses and midwives. *Nursing Open, 10*(12), 7585–7595. https://doi.org/10.1002/nop2.2017

Kessler, R. C., Aguilar-Gaxiola, S., Alonso, J., Benjet, C., Bromet, E. J., Cardoso, G., Degenhardt, L., de Girolamo, G., Dinolova, R. V., Ferry, F., Florescu, S., Gureje, O., Haro, J. M., Huang, Y., Karam, E. G., Kawakami, N., Lee, S., Lepine, J. P., Levinson, D., Navarro-Mateu, F., Pennell, B. E., Piazza, M., Posada-Villa, J., Scott, K. M., Stein, D. J., Ten Have, M., Torres, Y., Viana, M. C., Petukhova, M. V., Sampson, N. A., Zaslavsky, A. M., & Koenen, K. C. (2017). Trauma and PTSD in the WHO World Mental Health Surveys. *European Journal of Psychotraumatology, 8*(Suppl 5), 1353383. https://doi.org/10.1080/20008198.2017.1353383

Kimberg, L., & Wheeler, M. (2019). Trauma and trauma-informed care. In M. Gerber (Ed.), *Trauma-informed healthcare approaches.* Springer.

King, L. A., & Hicks, J. A. (2021). The science of meaning in life. *Annual Review of Psychology, 72,* 561–584. https://doi.org/10.1146/annurev-psych-072420-122921

Kira, I. (2021). The development-based taxonomy of stressors and traumas: An initial empirical validation. *Psychology, 12*(10), 1575–1614. https://doi.org/10.4236/psych.2021.121009

Kira, I. A. (2022). Taxonomy of stressors and traumas: An update of the development-based trauma framework (DBTF): A life-course perspective on stress and trauma. *Traumatology, 28*(1), 84–97. https://doi.org/10.1037/trm0000305

Kira, I. A., Shuweikh, H., Al-Huwailiah, A., El-Wakeel, S. A., Waheep, N. N., Ebada, E. E., & Ibrahim, E. R. (2022). The direct and indirect impact of trauma types and cumulative stressors and traumas on executive functions. *Applied Neuropsychology, 29*(5), 1078–1094. https://doi.org/10.1080/23279095.2020.1848835

Kira, I. A., Shuweikh, H., Ashby, J. S., Elwakeel, S. A., Alhuwailah, A., Sous, M. S. F., Baali, S. B. A., Azdaou, C., Oliemat, E. M., & Jamil, H. J. (2023). The impact of COVID-19 traumatic stressors on mental health: Is COVID-19 a new trauma type. *International Journal of Mental Health and Addiction, 21*(1), 51–70. https://doi.org/10.1007/s11469-021-00577-0

Knight, C. (2019). Trauma-informed practice and care: Implications for field instruction. *Clinical Social Work Journal, 47*, 79–89. https://doi.org/10.1007/s10615-018-0661

Kolaitis, G., & Olff, M. (2017). Psychotraumatology in Greece. *European Journal of Psychotraumatology, 8*(Suppl 4), 135175. https://doi.org/10.1080/20008198.2017.1351757

Levenson, J. (2020). Translating trauma-informed principles into social work practice. *Social Work, 65*(3), 288–298. https://doi.org/10.1093/sw/swaa020

Levin-Aspenson, H. F., & Greene, A. L. (2024). Rethinking trauma-related psychopathology in the Hierarchical Taxonomy of Psychopathology (HiTOP). *Journal of Traumatic Stress*, 1–11. https://doi.org/10.1002/jts.23014

Louis-Dreyfus, J. (Host). (2023, April 25). Julia gets wise with Ruth Reichl. In *Wiser Than Me*. Lemonada.

Mittelmark, M. B., & Bauer, G. F. (2022). Salutogenesis as a theory, as an orientation and as the sense of coherence. In M. B. Mittelmark, G. F. Bauer, L. Vaandrager, J. M. Pelikan, S. Sagy, M. Eriksson, B. Lindström, & C. M. Magistretti (Eds.), *The handbook of salutogenesis* (2nd ed.; pp. 11–17). Springer Open.

Morgan-López, A. A., Saavedra, L. M., Hien, D. A., Norman, S. B., Fitzpatrick, S. S., Ye, A., Killeen, T. K., Ruglass, L. M., Blakey, S. M., & Back, S. E. (2023). Differential symptom weighting in estimating empirical threshold for underlying PTSD severity: Toward a "platinum" standard for diagnosis? *International Journal of Methods in Psychiatric Research, 32*(3), e1963. https://doi.org/10.1002/mpr.1963

Munjiza, J., Britvic, D., & Crawford, M. J. (2019). Lasting personality pathology following exposure to severe trauma in adulthood: Retrospective cohort study. *BMC Psychiatry, 19*(1), 3. https://doi.org/10.1186/s12888-018-1975-5

Nagata, D. K., Kim, J. H. J., & Gone, J. P. (2024). Intergenerational transmission of ethnoracial historical trauma in the United States. *Annual Review of Clinical Psychology, 20*. https://doi.org/10.1146/annurev-clinpsy-080822-044522

References

Park, C. L., Currier, J. M., Harris, J. I., & Slattery, J. M. (2017). *Trauma, meaning, and spirituality: Translating research into clinical practice*. American Psychological Association. https://doi.org/10.1037/15961-000

Purtle, J. (2018). Systematic review of evaluations of trauma-informed organizational interventions that include staff trainings. *Trauma, Violence, & Abuse, 21*(4), 725–740. https://doi.org/10.1177/1524838018791304

Quiñones, M., Gold, S. N., & Ellis, A. (2022). Chapter 3 – Defining trauma, adversity, & toxic stress. In A. N. Marsh and L. J. Cox (Ed.), *Not just bad kids: The adversity and disruptive behavior link* (pp. 67–93). Academic Press.

Robinson, L., Smith, M. A., & Segal, J. (2023). Emotional and psychological trauma. https://www.helpguide.org/articles/ptsd-trauma/coping-with-emotional-and-psychological-trauma.htm

Rubin, D. C., Boals, A., & Hoyle, R. H. (2014). Narrative centrality and negative affectivity: Independent and interactive contributors to stress reactions. *Journal of Experimental Psychology: General, 143*, 1159–1170. https://doi.org/10.1037/a0035165

Schäfer, S. K., Becker, N., King, L., Horsch, A., & Michael, T. (2019). The relationship between sense of coherence and posttraumatic stress: A meta-analysis. *European Journal of Psychotraumatology, 10*(1), 1562839. https://doi.org/10.1080/20008198.2018.1562839

Schimmenti, A. (2017). The trauma factor: Examining the relationships among different types of trauma, dissociation, and psychopathology. *Journal of Trauma & Dissociation, 19*(5), 552–571. https://doi.org/10.1080/15299732.2017.1402400

Scull, A. (2022). *Desperate remedies: Psychiatry's turbulent quest to cure mental illness*. Belknap Press.

Spytska, L. (2023). Psychological trauma and its impact on a person's life prospects. *Scientific Bulletin of Mukachevo State University. Series, 9*(3), 82–90. https://doi.org/10.52534/msu-pp3.2023.82

Starcevic, A. (Ed.). (2019). *Psychological trauma*. Intech Open.

Substance Abuse and Mental Health Services Administration (SAMHSA). (2014). *SAMHSA's concept of trauma and guidance for a trauma-informed approach* [pdf file]. Substance Abuse and Mental Health Services Administration.

Sweeton, J. (2019). *Trauma treatment toolbox*. PESI Publishing.

Szczygiel, P. (2018). On the value and meaning of trauma-informed practice: Honoring safety, complexity, and relationship. *Smith College Studies in Social Work, 88*(2), 115–134. https://doi.org/10.1080/00377317.2018.1438006

Tedeschi, R. G., & Calhoun, L. G. (1995). *Trauma & transformation: Growing in the aftermath of suffering*. Sage Publications, Inc.

Tedeschi, R. G., Shakespeare-Finch, J., Taku, K., & Calhoun, L. G. (2018). *Posttraumatic growth: Theory, research, and applications*. Routledge.

Terr, L. C. (1991). Childhood traumas: An outline and overview. *American Journal of Psychiatry*, *148*, 10–20. https://doi.org/10.1176/ajp.148.1.10

Tomlinson, C. A., Shin, S. H., Burton, C., & Jiskrova, G. K. (2024). Patterns of adverse childhood experience and mental health symptoms among young adults. *Child and Youth Services Review*, Article 107680. https://doi.org/10.1016/j.childyouth.2024.107680

U.S. Department of Veterans Affairs National Center for PTSD (VA). (2024). Common reactions after trauma. https://www.ptsd.va.gov/understand/isitptsd/common_reactions.asp

Yang, L., Liu, S., & Lin, R. (2020). The role of light in regulating seed dormancy and germination. *Journal of Integrative Plant Biology*, *62*(9), 1310–1326. https://doi.org/10.1111/jipb.13001

References

Chapter Two
The Neurobiology of Trauma

Overview

Trauma is a life-threatening event that has a profound impact on a person's life and health, depending on the trauma, the intensity, length of the event, recurrences, episodic events, or ongoing trauma. The neurobiology of trauma and resilience is a recent research focus. Chapter 2: The Neurobiology of Trauma focuses on the current understanding of how trauma affects people and the impact of trauma on the human body. A variety of factors trigger traumatic symptoms, including physical, emotional, and mental health issues. The study of the neurobiology of traumatic stress has evolved from the view that trauma is a maladaptive reaction to a broader view of how stress and trauma impact brain functioning, personality, and relationships. Included in Chapter 2 is a discussion of the contemporary use of polyvagal theory, the braking system that reduces the threat of harm, and the utility of neuroception and interoception. Finally, resilience is explored in its vital role in emotion regulation and trauma recovery.

Stress

Stress comes in varying ways to people. For example, Jim and Brenda have experienced tense situations, but each has responded differently. Here are their stories. Jim, a 34-year-old married man, never realized how stressful life could be. He grew up in a safe home, receiving support in academics and activities. Jim landed his first job after attending college with a substantial scholarship. He married his college sweetheart and found a job that paid well. Jim and his wife Amy held full-time positions. The first

DOI: 10.4324/9781003463009-2

five years were terrific. They were expecting their first child and soon learned the child might have some difficulties. This turn of events required numerous physician visits, hospitalizations, and an early delivery at six months. During this time, Jim and Amy built a house, choosing all the materials and scheduling a move amid the problematic pregnancy. Additional stress occurred when they had problems navigating family relationships. Jim experienced high blood pressure, sleep disturbance, and constant worry. Some relationships became so demanding that he began to cut people out of his life. While Jim had plenty of friends and family, his estrangement from some who once supported him bothered him.

Brenda's life had stress earlier on. She described memories from childhood, including the taste of cold, fresh milk full of rich flavor, friends laughing as they would climb on playground equipment, rolling on a grassy hill, or sledding down a snowy bank. She recalled the smell of apple pie baking in the oven or the taste of soda pop that her grandma gave her. Brenda yearns to return to those moments when life was fun, exciting, and peaceful, free of worry. However, life was difficult as she lived in poverty with divorced parents, sharing a two-bedroom house with another family, and struggling to make ends meet. Her mother worked hard at her job, but she was not available to ensure the children's safety, which meant Brenda's father was free to come and take the children away without their mother's permission. Brenda's life was stressful and frightening, which contributed to her lifelong battle with anxiety. While Brenda's family had moments of pleasure and joy, she faced a worrisome and unstable life. As an adult, Brenda's struggle with food and financial insecurity continued despite having a good income.

Stress is a natural part of living, and while it can drive performance, increase motivation, or move us toward a goal, it can also become a burden. The degree to which individuals can bear stress is called allostatic load. The concept, introduced by McEwen and Stellar (1993), refers to the cost of ongoing stress (Guidi et al., 2020). Allostatic overload occurs because of frequent exposure to stressful situations, resulting in physiological arousal, difficulty adapting to re-occurring stressors, an inability to decrease or end the physiological hyperarousal, or insufficient resources to manage the encumbrance (Guidi et al., 2020).

The American Psychological Association conducts an annual survey on stress in America, distributed to thousands of adults in the United States. According to the 2023 report, 58% of Americans have chronic health conditions, and 45% report a mental health disorder (APA, 2024). This rise represents an increase of 10% in health conditions and a 14% increase in mental illness from 2019 (APA, 2024). Mid-career adults report that finances and the economy are the factors causing the most significant burden. Approximately 24% of Americans report a stress level between 8 and 10 on a scale of one to 10, with 1 being no stress and 10 being the highest stress level (APA, 2024). Strain is no stranger among the U.S. population, yet people in other countries report more significant stress. In a 2021–2022 survey of adults in 34 countries, stress was one of the biggest health concerns. Argentina, Switzerland, and South Korea report that more than one-third of the population believes emotional strain is a significant problem (Vankar, 2023).

Think for a moment about stress. What things are most stressful for you? When it comes, what do you experience in your body or emotions? Do you push your thoughts and feelings away? Does your reaction differ with varying levels of stress? How do you manage it? The demands we experience daily may vary, but the ubiquity of stress is familiar. Considering how these pressures affect the human body provides a further understanding of how trauma affects people.

The Brain's Response to Perceived Stress

MacLean's studies of the brain summarized how the brain responded to stressful circumstances (MacLean, 1988). His work hypothesized the triune brain, meaning the cortex (neomammalian), limbic system (paleomammalian), and brainstem (reptilian), whose roles comprise thinking, emoting, and surviving (Miller-Karas, 2023). The cortex controls executive functioning, which includes logic, decision-making, learning, memory, and inhibitory functions (Herry & Johansen, 2014). The limbic system and midbrain handle emotions and relay information, while the brain stem supports survival instincts and autonomic processes, such as breathing (Rosenthal, 2019). This concept spurred further study of the interactive processes in the brain in stress response, which includes the function of the human nervous system. The human nervous system keeps people alive through two primary systems: the brain and spinal cord's central nervous system and the autonomic nervous system. The sympathetic nervous system, part of the autonomic nervous system, protects the human body during stressful moments (LeDoux & Pine, 2016).

The body survives by continually adapting to internal and external stimuli to maintain homeostasis or a stable operating system. This equilibrium is maintained through the central nervous and autonomic nervous systems as hormones are released to mediate imbalances in the system (O'Connor et al., 2021). Under stress, the brain receives sensory information through the amygdala, which interprets the stimuli as a system threat based on novel information and previous experience. The amygdala, part of the limbic system, is associated with fear conditioning and negative and positive learning. This perceived danger triggers a subcortical, sensorimotor response and cortical, cognitive awareness and appraisal of the perceived threat (LeDoux & Pine, 2016). This reaction stimulates the sympathetic nervous system for a defensive reaction. When heightened, the sympathetic nervous system works with the hypothalamus–pituitary–adrenal (HPA) axis, a neuroendocrinological pathway, to release hormones called catecholamines, such as adrenaline and noradrenaline and cortisol, to increase body energy (Stephens & Wand, 2012). With the sympathetic nervous system activated, the heart rate and blood pressure surge to supply blood to the extremities, the hands, and feet for fighting or fleeing. The pupils dilate, and salivation decreases. This defensive response lasts a short duration to protect the body and transitions to parasympathetic recovery, promoting energy conservation and a more tranquil state (Ford & Courtois, 2020).

Nurture Understanding

Think about what you have learned about stress and the brain. If you had to explain how the brain responds to stress, how could you say it briefly, accurately, and clearly? We describe it to clients in the following way. Imagine you enter a room, and there is a hungry tiger. You can see its jaws dripping saliva, hear its chest rumbling, and smell it even though you are across the room. In seconds, your heart begins to race, and you begin to shake because your senses have detected a potential threat. You feel frozen because there is no one around to help. Instantly, a surge of energy occurs in your body, and you run, knowing you cannot fight this fierce animal.

As you run down the hall, you notice you have boundless energy, moving faster than ever with the sharpest vision. Your ability to weave through the hall and around doors until you reach safety is unsurpassed. As you run into a room where you can close the door, you lift desks and chairs and pile them in front, blocking anyone or anything from entering. You have just experienced activation of your sympathetic nervous system in response to the tiger.

It happened quickly and without your willpower. You had no opportunity to think, choose, or decide. Your body did what it needed to do in the moment for your survival. That happens when your senses send signals to the amygdala, the threat detector.

The amygdala sends a warning to the hypothalamus, which then transmits it to the pituitary gland, commanding the release of adrenaline and cortisol. These processes cause your heart to beat more quickly, your eyesight to sharpen, and increased oxygen to your extremities to strengthen them. However, they also shut down your digestive system and short-circuit your thinking brain. This is the body's way of protecting itself. After the event, you find yourself exhausted but able to move to a relaxed state. This is the effect of stress.

- Is it possible to remove stress?
- How might some stress be helpful to people?

Traumatic Stress

As mentioned in Chapter 1, different trauma experiences have varied effects on individuals, families, and groups. The complexity of trauma makes it more challenging to determine the etiology or the causes behind traumatic symptoms. Trauma-related stress disorders, such as PTSD, have established criteria, but not all symptoms are exhibited by every individual (Burback et al., 2024). Among those exposed to or affected by disturbing events, the risk factors include personal predisposition, genetic and epigenetic sequences, environmental influences, and physiological responses (Daskalakis et al., 2018). Knowing the various components that contribute to symptom development is crucial. A general knowledge of trauma etiology informs those desiring to collaborate with people.

For example, studies of sex differences in PTSD show females are twice as likely to develop traumatic stress symptoms as males because of differences in sex-related hormones (Tolin & Foa, 2006). Other studies show sex differences in the stress response at the molecular level, receptor levels, and biomarkers (Yehuda et al., 2015). A study with over 500 women with trauma exposure showed differences between White and racial minority women, with African American and Latina women at greater risk of developing PTSD. This difference could relate to elevated baselines of physiological arousal because of chronic micro- and macro-aggressions faced by ethnic minorities (Ruglass et al., 2020). These examples help trauma workers understand the risk, prevalence, and symptom appearance among different individuals. However, all people experiencing stress or trauma share similar physical responses to taxing conditions.

The Fear Continuum

The discoveries of neuroscience have enhanced the contribution to a broader view of traumatic stress. In the past, individuals with symptoms were viewed as psychopathological, exhibiting maladaptive reactions to stress or decreased adaptive reflexivity (Ford & Courtois, 2020). This view led to further stigmatization of people who have a mental health disorder. With neurobiology, this perspective shifted to recognize stress responses as adaptive to surmounting distress.

One of the first changes occurred when recognizing that fear conditioning precipitated the development of disturbing reactions. Watson and Rayner uncovered this in their study of Little Albert, which is now considered an unethical experiment. Their study of Little Albert discovered they could teach a person to fear an object by pairing a conditioned stimulus with an aversive unconditioned stimulus (Watson & Rayner, 1920). Subsequently, Estes and Skinner conducted experiments on rats to condition stress responses, demonstrating that fear-based mechanisms could be involved in mental health disorders, such as specific phobias and PTSD (Estes & Skinner, 1941). In 1961, Wolpe hypothesized that undoing the fear conditioning required systematic desensitization, which combined relaxation with correction of cognitive appraisals. Exposure therapy came from this research, wherein therapists worked to extinguish conditioned responses of panic and anxiety. However, the memories surrounding the conditioning situation did not disappear, and when a person was vulnerable, the fear responses returned (Maren & Holmes, 2016). While these experiments led to further understanding of anxiety or stress responses, these were inadequate to address human conditions of fear and the resulting symptoms. Observing and describing behaviors, conditioning, or reconditioning behaviors were just the beginning. The study of traumatic responses and the treatment required a look inside the brain.

Cultivate Knowledge

As you read about the fear circuit, can you think of a time when you were a child and had a fearful experience? Does that still bother you today? Has that changed how you respond to anything? For example, as a child, Harry remembered visiting the zoo. He was excited to see the animals and wore his favorite red hat. He hoped the hat would allow animals to notice him and come close so he could pet a few. While he was there, they stopped by the tiger's cage. Harry ventured near the plexiglass wall.

The tiger appeared to be resting. Suddenly, the tiger stood and faced Harry. He moved his head closer to the wall, which frightened Harry. While Harry was safe, he did not feel so. He jumped, and his hat fell off. From that point forward, Harry was afraid to wear his hat. As an adult, Harry often stated how much he hated anything red. Now it is your turn.

- How were you conditioned?
- What is one unconditioned response that became tied to an unconditioned stimulus?
- In Harry's story, what is the conditioned stimulus?

Brain Areas Affected by Trauma

Traumatic events can overwhelm the body's systems, depending on the trauma, the intensity, length of the event, recurrences, episodic events, or ongoing trauma. Sweeton (2019) states five main brain areas related to trauma: the fear center, the interoception center, the memory center, the thinking center, and the self-regulation center. The fear center is related to the amygdala, the interoception center relates to the insula, the hippocampus is the memory center, the prefrontal cortex, or the front of the brain, is the thinking center and the anterior cingulate cortex is the system's self-regulation center (Sweeton, 2019). Understanding how trauma affects each center guides helpers in responding appropriately and choosing helpful interventions.

The Amygdala

The amygdala, in the limbic system, is the fear center, and its purpose is to detect threats from the external environment and internal sensations from the body. It alerts the hypothalamus of the potential danger, which activates a response in the pituitary gland, followed by a release of hormones from the adrenal glands. This activation in the fear center allows an individual to mobilize resources, resulting in a flight, fight, or freeze response to protect the individual. When a person has post-trauma symptoms, the fear center is over-activated, which causes one to be hypervigilant and over-reactive to non-threatening situations (Sweeton, 2019; Sweeton, 2022).

With trauma, a person's brain may change. The amygdala may enlarge (Keefe et al., 2022). Biological changes cause system dysregulation with an overstimulated amygdala (Rosenthal, 2019). Individuals with PTSD experience heightened activation in association with the amygdala (McLaughlin et al., 2014). Among people diagnosed with PTSD, the sympathetic nervous system shows an autonomic hyperarousal response that is higher than those people without a PTSD diagnosis (Zoladz & Diamond, 2016). People with a chronic stress condition may become sensitized to stimuli, interpreting neutral faces as aggressive, fearful faces as angry, and responding with shame to smiling faces (Bardeen & Orcutt, 2011; Steuwe et al., 2014). This dysregulation causes individuals to perceive nonexistent threats, leading to disrupted communication between body systems, heightened limbic arousal, diminished cognitive functioning, and prolonged sympathetic nervous system activation (Nicholson et al., 2017).

The Insula

The insular cortex, located deep in the lateral sulcus, has multiple functions (Uddin et al., 2017). Sweeton (2019) states that the anterior insula is the interoception and proprioception center. This part of the brain enables a person to maintain a sense of balance and spatial orientation, as well as to decipher internal experiences and connect those with internal sensations (Sweeton, 2019). The insula serves as a communication hub, specifically with the amygdala. The anterior insula also functions as a center communicating with the auditory and visual systems. With trauma, repeated activation of the bilateral anterior insula may occur, which results in hyperarousal and re-experiencing the trauma (Leroy et al., 2022). Another type of functioning associated with this region is self–other distinction, which is implicated in dissociative experiences (Sperduti et al., 2011). After a traumatic experience, the insular cortex may become underactive, making it difficult for a person to connect their inner sensations. They might lose the ability to ascertain if a situation is occurring in the present or past. This change can lead to flashbacks of numbness or apathy (Sweeton, 2022).

The Hippocampus

When overwhelmed, the brain responds with adaptive alterations in executive functioning memory systems, changes in architecture, shrinkage of the hippocampus, and decreased communication between the hippocampus and the salience network used for learning (Keefe et al., 2022). Further biological changes cause an underactive hippocampus in reactive mode and a continuous elevation of stress hormones, leading to

Brain Areas Affected by Trauma

fatigue (Rosenthal, 2019). Chronic stress reduces gray matter in the prefrontal cortex, which may lead to increased impulsivity and loss of delayed gratification (Schauer & Elbert, 2010). The hippocampus functions as the memory center, organizing memories as they occur. After trauma, the shrinking hippocampus affects memory recall and the ability to feel safe (Herry & Johansen, 2014; Sweeton, 2019).

In studies of the hippocampus, which is responsible for memory consolidation, spatial context, and learning, traumatic stress may impact memory coding and recall and result in reduced volume. Trauma may affect a person's ability to practice neuroception or detect safe environments (Banks, 2016). Chronic stress reduces gray matter in the prefrontal cortex, which may lead to increased impulsivity and loss of delayed gratification (Schauer & Elbert, 2010). These physical changes in brain functioning affect a person's personality, way of thinking, behaviors, and relationships.

The Prefrontal Cortex

The prefrontal cortex is the part of the brain responsible for logic, reasoning, and decision-making; in other words, the thinking center. The prefrontal cortex also plays a significant role in determining threat, inhibiting threat, and emotion regulation (Kredlow et al., 2022). Emotion regulation involves the sensitivity to intense emotions and modulating the system's response. The prefrontal cortex regulates emotion using bidirectional communication with subcortical areas, such as the amygdala and anterior cingulate cortex. Severe or repeated trauma can cause molecular changes in this circuitry, producing adverse long-term effects (Kredlow et al., 2022; Weis et al., 2022). These molecular changes may cause reduced gray matter and decreased connectivity between the prefrontal cortex and subcortical regions. This change can lead to emotion dysregulation and increased impulsivity (Theodoratou et al., 2023). Changes may also contribute to decreased concentration and difficulty in decision-making (Sweeton, 2022).

The Anterior Cingulate Cortex

The self-regulation center, which involves the prefrontal cortex and the anterior cingulate cortex, is vital for daily functioning (Sweeton, 2019). The anterior cingulate cortex encodes emotions, focusing on negative ones such as anxiety, fear, and anger, and aids in regulating amygdala activity (Liberati & Perrotta, 2024). When over-activated,

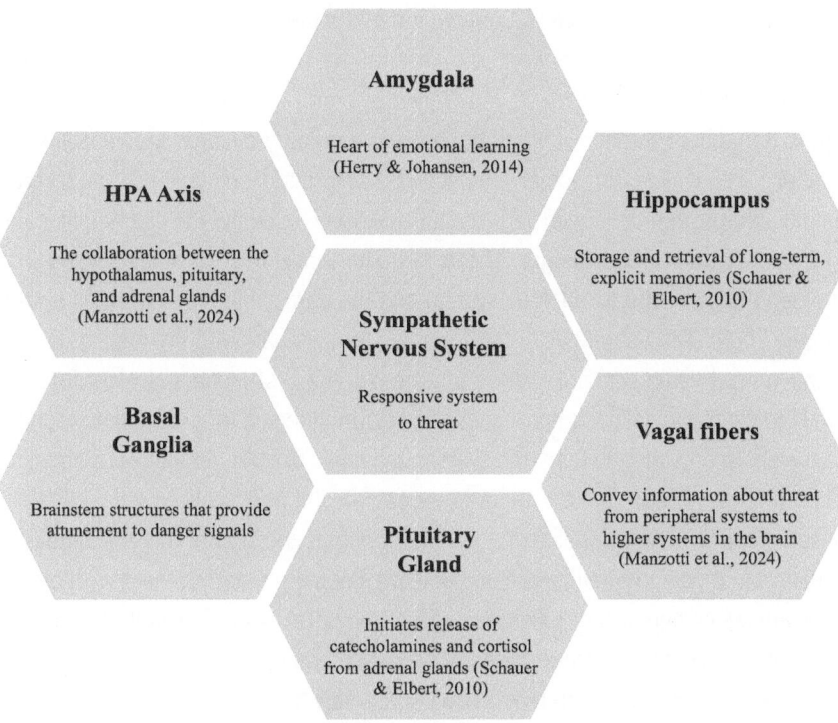

FIGURE 2.1 Brain Areas Affected by Trauma.

(Keefe et al., 2022; Kredlow et al., 2022; Liberati & Perrotta, 2024; McLaughlin et al., 2014; Nicholson et al., 2017; Rosenthal, 2019; Sweeton, 2019; Sweeton, 2022; Uddin et al., 2017; Zoladz & Diamond, 2016).

the result is increased cardiovascular and behavioral activity, heightened avoidance, and blunting positive reward-related motivation (Arnsten et al., 2023). Interestingly, some studies show that males, such as war veterans, may have reduced volume and hypofunctionality in this region. However, most studies indicate hyperactivity, which relates to persistent and intrusive memories and flashbacks (Liberati & Perrotta, 2024) (Figure 2.1).

Polyvagal Theory

The behavioral field turned to studies that explained what was happening and how to regain prior or new functioning levels to help people with physiological changes. While some studies were unrelated to trauma, they became seminal in new treatments for traumatic experiences by offering innovative information. One of these discoveries came when Porges (2009) identified the hierarchical system of the auto-nomic nervous system in his work with infants. He outlined how the vagus nerve, associated with cranial nerve X, ran from the brain, and connected with various organs throughout the body, highlighting its two primary circuits: the ventral vagal complex, responsible for social connectivity, emotional engagement, and verbal communication; and the dorsal vagal complex extending below the diaphragm, caus-ing immobilization amid danger. These systems work in a scaffolded framework between the sympathetic nervous system and the parasympathetic nervous system (Porges, 2009). The autonomic system readies for survival, with the highest priority on the ventral vagal complex. When threatened, the first instinct is a cry for help, using the ventral vagal complex or connection with others. If others are not around or are unable or unwilling to help, the system will move to fight or flight to re-establish safety (Porges, 2009). If the trauma is perpetual, the body will be immobilized to conserve energy. The emphasis of polyvagal theory is the central role the vagal sys-tem plays in a person's ability to communicate, cooperate, and connect with others, especially when under threat. Porges and Furman (2011) state the ventral vagal sys-tem is of significant concern in terms of how it can inhibit the sympathetic nervous system and the HPA axis, thereby allowing an individual to calm down, re-engage with people, and move to a parasympathetic state of recovery and rest. He described these branches of the parasympathetic nervous system as a type of braking system (Porges, 2009).

Critics of the polyvagal theory believe it places too much emphasis on the vagus nerve while ignoring other brain areas involved in processing stress and trauma, such as the amygdala, hypothalamus, insula, anterior cingulate cortex, and even the medulla (Bottaccioli & Bottaccioli, 2020). Some state that little evidence favors the connec-tions of the vagus nerve, as Porges suggests, or that the theory is accurate in its anatomical descriptions (Giroux et al., 2023; Manzotti et al., 2024). Nonetheless, the influence of the polyvagal theory in trauma-informed practice is significant. Porges offers a way to understand and explain the importance of safety via neuroception in trauma healing and growth. The theory helps to remove the shame and guilt that traumatized individuals experience in its explanation of autonomic processes in the body. Polyvagal theory offers a way to develop strategies that support people with traumatic experiences (Porges, 2024). This theory aligns with Van der Kolk et al.'s (2016) explanation of how trauma affects the body.

Threat Responses

Trauma stress produces a series of responses as mechanisms for action to reduce the threat of harm to the body: freeze, fight, flight, and tonic immobility (Fragkaki et al., 2016). These reactions to potential threats involve multiple interactions from the autonomic system, behavioral responses, and endocrine changes (Signoret-Genest et al., 2023). Some also consider additional stages, such as fright, flag, or fawn (Schwartz, 2016). The body undergoes these stages to protect and defend itself (Fragkaki et al., 2016). The initial reaction to traumatic stress is freezing, like an animal may freeze when sensing danger nearby. When this immobilization occurs, it allows the body to gather the energy needed for action. An individual's physical energy increases as physiological arousal increases. Freezing is not a passive state, however. This freezing allows an individual the opportunity to decide their response to the threat (Livermore et al., 2022). However, freezing may not resolve the current threat; the stress conditions continue or worsen. In that case, this can lead to a dissociative state, preoccupation with previous or future danger, intrusive thoughts, or memories resulting in rumination, negative alterations in beliefs of the world and people, and dysregulation of emotion, attention, behaviors, relatedness, and identity (Fragkaki et al., 2016).

Fight and flight reactions occur after the individual has analyzed their ability to neutralize the danger through physical action. Survival requires short bursts of energy, and if the person determines they cannot surmount the hazard, they will attempt to flee the situation. However, either action may cause further distress (Fragkaki et al., 2016). Tonic immobility may occur if the individual feels trapped. While the body initially responds with tachycardia, in this state, bradycardia, or a slower heart rate, may occur (Signoret-Genest et al., 2023). Signs of immobility include somatoform responses, exhibited by paralysis or blindness, or psychoform responses, including depersonalization, derealization, fugue states, or psychogenic amnesias. Other examples of immobility include altered beliefs, involuntary avoidance, emotional numbness, detachment from relationships, shame or guilt, and difficulty with goal-oriented behavior (Fragkaki et al., 2016) (Figure 2.2).

Neuroception and Interoception

As the biology of trauma progresses, so does the knowledge of treatment opportunities. When one considers that threat, or perceived threat, galvanizes the sympathetic

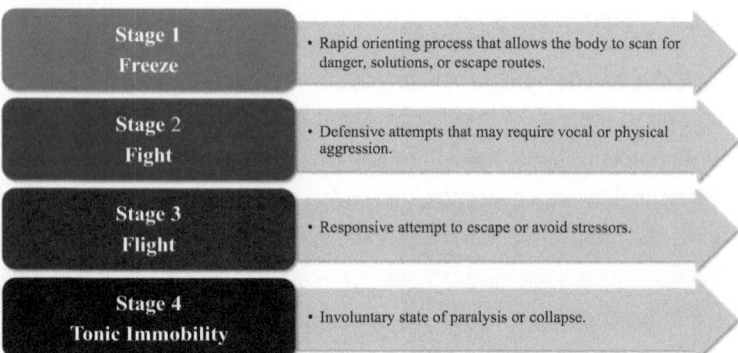

FIGURE 2.2   Threat Responses.

(Fragkaki et al., 2016).

nervous system, part of the treatment protocol changes to focus on how people perceive stress and can maintain physical and emotional homeostasis under the most challenging circumstances. As mentioned earlier, neuroception becomes a key component in healing, interoception, or the perception and awareness of bodily sensations (Price & Hooven, 2018).

The Assessment of Threat

The body's ability to detect threats or neuroception is needed for survival. The continuous activation of the sympathetic nervous system impairs an individual's capacity to discern between safety and danger. One common occurrence among children who experience neglect or abuse is feeling more endangered, even in situations with no jeopardy (Gerge, 2020). This perceptive ability changes because of brain activity and altered architecture from repeated traumatic episodes (Teicher & Samson, 2016). This inability to discern safety interferes with emotion regulation, essential in reducing tension, hyperarousal, and changing negative attributions. It may elicit rigid response patterns, which is counterproductive for the sufferer (Fonagy & Luyten, 2016). According to Van der Kolk et al. (2016), many people's brains are conditioned to fear based on their traumatic encounters. While the physiological process is yet unknown, some researchers theorize this occurs through accelerated information processing, which collapses the current situation into overwhelming past unintegrated experiences. If true, this means an individual loses the ability to discriminate whether a situation is safe or a dysfunctional capacity for neuroception (Gerge, 2020). Treatment must include the re-development of this skill, which may occur through increasing interoceptive awareness.

Interoceptive Awareness

The perception of internal sensations requires one to attune to the inner states of their body, such as awareness of one's heartbeat, breathing, sense of fullness at eating, and emotional states. Interoceptive awareness connects to emotion regulation and managing distressing emotions (Craig, 2015). Interoception requires communication between the body and cortical oversight or the process by which the cognitive centers in the brain interpret the information received. Sensations underlie most emotions, especially intense ones. With interoceptive awareness, the individual can identify, monitor, and respond healthily to these internal messages (Craig, 2015). Therefore, understanding and increasing interoceptive awareness helps people regulate intense emotional reactions. By accurately interpreting sensations, regulation strategies can reduce physiological reactions to stress or trauma, improving well-being. These strategies help the sympathetic nervous system to down-regulate, becoming less sensitive and reactive to cues, which decreases posttraumatic stress symptoms (Price & Hooven, 2018). This process enables an individual to live life more fully when not disturbed by the uncomfortable physical and psychological effects of trauma.

Tending Your Technique

There are several ways to teach others about these two concepts. First, to help people understand neuroception, we show them there is a difference between being physically safe and feeling emotionally safe. One way to do that is by asking the following question: "Are you 100% physically safe right now?"

People with a trauma history are likely to respond no because they perceive danger. They do not feel emotionally safe – ever. We must help them grasp their physical safety before moving them to understanding emotional safety. Once they are ready, then we can say, "The reason you do not feel safe is because your past painful experiences are intruding in the present moment, and that trauma is causing you to perceive danger when there is no physical danger right now." Practicing this skill throughout the day and assessing the difference between physical and emotional safety will rebuild neuroception.

Polyvagal Theory

To build interoception, we ask clients to do a 2–3-second task every time they drink water. Then, we ask them to do a body scan, yawn, hold and release a muscle, or some other quick activity that makes them pay attention to their body. We ask them to describe the experience. Doing this numerous times reconnects them to their body, increasing their inner awareness.

A Flourishing Focus

Adopting a salutogenic evaluation that focuses on a person's use of internal and external resources encourages and motivates people. Resilience is a concept that researchers have varying interpretations of, encompassing traits, processes, and outcomes (Southwick et al., 2014). It involves external factors and internal resources (Ahern et al., 2006). External factors may include family, friends, or other social support systems, while internal factors include personality, traits, or coping styles. The encouragement of resiliency brings hope to those who bear difficulties.

One of the first lessons counselors learn in training is that providing hope is vital in therapy. Hope theory describes hope as a two-dimensional cognitive activity that involves one's capacity to start and maintain purposeful action and the ability to find a practical course of action (Snyder, 1994). Hope studies show a positive correlation between well-being among those who face adversity, a sense of empowerment, increased self-control, and optimism (Hellman & Gwinn, 2017; Munoz et al., 2017). When working with traumatized individuals, helpers can highlight moments when people transcend their dire circumstances, choosing to rely on outer resources and inner strengths. Bringing attention to this enhances the survivors' resilience.

Resilience is a multidimensional construct that reveals the influence of genetics, epigenetics, development, psychosocial environment, psychological precipitants, neurochemical processes, and pharmacological effects (Friedberg & Malefakis, 2022). The study of resilience neurobiology is novel. Resilience relates to a person's ability to adapt amid challenges and life disruptions. A common misunderstanding is that resilient people are always positive and do not experience negative cognitions or emotions. Resilience is using positive coping strategies and optimism to balance negative experiences (Vindevogel et al., 2015).

People mistakenly consider that resilience is a pre-existing characteristic that is either present or not. Various people during COVID-19 emphasized resilience and advised medical providers, teachers, and other frontline workers to possess it. Unfortunately, this made these professionals believe the public viewed them as needing more resilience. This notion is problematic. All people have resilience, which changes over time according to different circumstances and is part of the neurobiological response to stress (Roeckner et al., 2021). When describing resilience to others, we use the metaphor of strengthening a muscle. The more one exercises, the stronger it grows.

From a neurobiological perspective, resilience is affected by changes in varied neural circuits. The discovery of interventions that enhance resilience uncovered the role of β-catenin, a protein found in the central nervous system. It mediates effects in the nucleus accumbens, the brain's reward region (Dias et al., 2015). Resilience involves the HPA axis, oxytocin pathways, serotonin transporters, and brain-derived neurotrophic factors (Vialou et al., 2010). In addition, neuroendocrine studies show the endocrine system's role in resilience (Feder et al., 2010). The implications of these studies may lead to enhanced therapeutic interventions. Indeed, the studies of the neurobiology of trauma and resilience offer more hope that recovery can occur for everyone.

To comprehend hope, investigators have identified neuroanatomic correlates of hope, one of which is the hippocampus, which seems to moderate hopefulness (Gondi et al., 2014). In studies of people with a cancer diagnosis, hope is independent of the clinical state or prognosis. Rustøen et al. (2011) performed a successful study of eight sessions to increase hope among patients with breast cancer. Other studies link hope with the prefrontal cortex, given that hope is a cognitive process. Researchers discovered a positive relationship between gray matter in the brain and hope in the first study of dispositional hope, the tendency to apply a cognitive-focused practice, including the plan to set, meet, and attain goals. Disposition hope may predict an individual's subjective well-being. People without hope had less gray matter in the left supplementary motor area. The findings from this study may foster further research into interventions that facilitate hope cultivation (Wang et al., 2020).

Gather Self-Awareness

- As you reflect on stressful experiences, can you identify how those affected your mind, emotions, and body?
- As clients or patients describe their trauma, what do you notice occurs internally for you?

A Flourishing Focus

- What thoughts, activities, or other things have you done to increase your resilience?

Chapter Summary

Chapter 2 explored traumatic stress, its impact on human health, and the contemporary understanding of trauma's neurobiological underpinnings. It began by discussing stress and its impact on individuals, with examples of Jim and Brenda, highlighting the concept of allostatic load. The American Psychological Association's survey on stress in America underscores the prevalence of chronic health conditions and mental health disorders due to stress. The brain's response to perceived stress is detailed, explaining the role of different brain areas and their impact on the body's physiological reactions. The concept of polyvagal theory, neuroception, and interoception was introduced, emphasizing their role in understanding, and treating trauma. The chapter discussed the fear continuum, traumatic stress, and the body's threat responses.

Furthermore, it explained the threat and interoceptive awareness assessment, shedding light on their importance in trauma treatment. Chapter 2 explored the concept of resilience, focusing on its multifaceted nature, emphasizing its internal and external components, and the role of hope in fostering resilience. The chapter also discussed strategies for increasing resilience and the neurobiological correlates of resilience, offering hope for recovery from trauma. Chapter 2 underscored the importance of hope and the neurobiological correlates of hope in trauma recovery. Overall, the chapter offered valuable insights into the neurobiological aspects of trauma and resilience, providing a foundation for trauma-informed practice and interventions.

Chapter Review

Please respond to the following questions.

1. What is the focus of Chapter 2?
2. What factors are discussed about trauma?
3. How does the brain respond to perceived stress in trauma?
4. How is the concept of resilience explored in the chapter?

Key Term Assessment

Review the following terms and try to explain each concept.

- Trauma response network
- Polyvagal theory
- Neuroception
- Interoception
- Resilience

Resources

The following resources may be helpful. At the time of this writing, they were accessible through the links provided.

- The National Institute for the Clinical Application of Behavioral Medicine (NICABM) offers webinars and workshops on the neurobiology of trauma. You can find the information here: https://www.nicabm.com/program/brain-trauma/
- The Polyvagal Institute is a non-profit organization dedicated to the development of novel paradigms for health and wellness. It provides training, community, and research, specifically related to Polyvagal Theory and the work of Dr. Stephen Porges. https://www.polyvagalinstitute.org
- The SAKI (Sexual Assault Kit Initiative) has a three-part webinar by psychology professor Rebecca Campbell that explains the neurobiology of sexual assault trauma. It is offered here: https://www.sakitta.org/toolkit/index.cfm?fuseaction=tool&tool=48

References

Ahern, N. R., Kiehl, E. M., Sole, M. L., & Byers, J. (2006). A review of instruments measuring resilience. *Issues in Comprehensive Pediatric Nursing, 29*, 103–125. https://doi.org/10.1080/01460860600677643

American Psychological Association. (2024). *Stress in America 2023: A nation recovering from collective trauma*. https://www.apa.org/news/press/releases/stress/2023/collective-trauma-recovery

Arnsten, A. F. T., Joyce, M. K. P., & Roberts, A. C. (2023). The aversive lens: Stress effects on the prefrontal-cingulate cortical pathways that regulate emotion. *Neuroscience & Biobehavioral Reviews*, *145*, 105000. https://doi.org/10.1016/j.neubiorev.2022.105000

Banks, A. (2016). *Wired to connect: The surprising link between brain science and strong, healthy relationships*. Penguin.

Bardeen, J. R., & Orcutt, H. K. (2011). Attentional control as a moderator of the relationship between posttraumatic stress symptoms and attentional threat bias. *Journal of Anxiety Disorders*, *25*(8), 1008–1018. https://doi.org/10.1016.j.janxdis.2011.06.009

Bottaccioli, F., & Bottaccioli, A. G. (2020). *Psycho neuro endocrine immunology and the science of the integrated care—the manual*. Edra.

Burback, L., Brémault-Phillips, S., Nijdam, M. J., McFarlane, A., & Vermetten, E. (2024). Treatment of posttraumatic stress disorder: A state-of-the-art review. *Current Neuropharmacology*, *22*, 557–635. https://doi.org/10.2174/1570159X21666230428091433

Craig, A. D. (2015). *How do you feel? An interoceptive moment with your neurobiological self*. Princeton University Press. https://doi.org/10.1515/9781400852727

Daskalakis, N. P., Rijal, C. M., King, C., Huckins, L. M., & Ressler, K. J. (2018). Recent genetics and epigenetics approaches to PTSD. *Current Psychiatry Reports*, *20*(5), 30. https://doi.org/10.1007/s11920-018-0898-7

Dias, M., Peltonen, K., Qouta, S. R., Palosaari, E., & Punamäki, R. (2015). Effectiveness of psychosocial intervention enhancing resilience among war-affected children and the moderating role of family factors. *Child Abuse and Neglect*, *40*, 24–35. https://doi.org/10.1016/j.chiabu.2014.12.002

Estes, W. K., & Skinner, B. F. (1941). Some quantitative properties of anxiety. *Journal of Experimental Psychology*, *29*(5), 390–400. https://doi.org/10.1037/h0062283

Feder, A., Nestler, E. J., Westphal, M., & Charney, D. S. (2010). Psychobiological mechanisms of resilience to stress. In J. W. Reich, A. J. Zautra, J. S. Hall, J. W. Reich, A. J. Zautra, & J. S. Hall (Eds.), *Handbook of adult resilience* (pp. 35–54). The Guilford Press.

Fonagy, P., & Luyten, P. (2016). A multilevel perspective on the development of borderline personality disorder (ch. 17). In D. Cicchetti (Ed.), *Developmental psychopathology: Maladaptation and psychopathology* (3rd ed., pp. 726–792). John Wiley & Sons, Inc. https://doi.org/10.1002/9781119125556.devpsy317

Ford, J. D., & Courtois, C. A. (Eds.). (2020). *Treating complex traumatic stress disorders in adults: Scientific foundations and therapeutic models* (2nd ed.). The Guilford Press.

Fragkaki, I., Thomas, K., & Sijbrandij, M. (2016). Posttraumatic stress disorder under ongoing threat: A review of neurobiological and neuroendocrine findings. *European Journal of Psychotraumatology*, *7*, Article 30915. https://doi.org/10.3402/ejpt.v7.30915

Friedberg, A., & Malefakis, D. (2022). Resilience, trauma and coping. *Psychodynamic Psychiatry*, *50*(2), 382–409. https://doi.org/10.1521/pdps.2022.50.2.382

Gerge, A. (2020). What neuroscience and neurofeedback can teach psychotherapists in the field of complex trauma: Interoception, neuroception and the embodiment of unspeakable events in treatment of complex PTSD, dissociative disorders and childhood traumatization. *Dissociation, 4*(3), 100164. https://doi.org/10.1016/j.ejtd.2020.100164

Giroux, C., Ahlers, D., & Miawotoe, A. (2023). Polyvagal approaches: Scientifically questionable but useful in practice. *Journal of Psychiatry Reform, 10*(11). https://journalofpsychiatryreform.com/2023/10/17/polyvagal-approaches-scientifically-questionable-but-useful-in-practice/

Gondi, V., Pugh, S. L., Tome, W. A., Caine, C., Corn, B., Kanner, A., Rowley, H., Kundapur, V., DeNittis, A., Greenspoon, J. N., Konski, A. A., Bauman, G. S., Shah, S., Shi, W., Wendland, M., Kachnic, L., & Mehta, M. P. (2014). Preservation of memory with conformal avoidance of the hippocampal neural stem-cell compartment during whole-brain radiotherapy for brain metastases (RTOG 0933): A phase II multi-institutional trial. *Journal of Clinical Oncology: Official Journal of the American Society of Clinical Oncology, 32*(34), 3810–3816. https://doi.org/10.1200/JCO.2014.57.2909

Guidi, J., Lucente, M., Sonino, N., & Fava, G. A. (2020). Allostatic load and its impact on health: A systematic review. *Psychotherapy and Psychosomatics, 90*(1), 11–27. https://doi.org/10.1159/000510696

Hellman, C. M., & Gwinn, C. (2017). Camp HOPE as an intervention for children exposed to domestic violence: A program evaluation of hope, and strength of character. *Child and Adolescent Social Work Journal, 34*, 269–276. https://doi.org/10.1007/s10902-012-9351-5

Herry, C., & Johansen, J. P. (2014). Encoding of fear learning and memory in distributed neuronal circuits. *Nature Neuroscience, 17*(12), 1644–1654. https://doi.org/10.1038/nn.3869

Keefe, J. R., Suarez-Jimenez, B., Zhu, X., Lazarov, A., Durosky, A., Such, A., Marohasy, C., Lissek, S., & Neria, Y. (2022). Elucidating behavioral and functional connectivity markers of aberrant threat discrimination in PTSD. *Depression and Anxiety, 39*(12), 891–901. https://doi.org/10.1002/da.23295

Kredlow, M. A., Fenster, R. J., Laurent, E. S., Ressler, K. J., & Phelps, E. A. (2022). Prefrontal cortex, amygdala, and threat processing: Implications for PTSD. *Neuropsychopharmacology, 47*, 247–259. https://doi.org/10.1013/s41386-021-01155-7

LeDoux, J. E., & Pine, D. S. (2016). Using neuroscience to help understand fear and anxiety: A two-system framework. *The American Journal of Psychiatry, 173*(11), 1083–1093. https://doi.org/10.1176/appi.ajp.2016.16030353

Leroy, A., Very, E., Birmes, P., Yger, P., Szaffarczyk, S., Lopes, R., Outteryck, O., Faure, C., Duhem, S., Grandgenèvre, P., Warembourg, F., Vaiva, G., & Jardri, R. (2022). Intrusive experiences in posttraumatic stress disorder: Treatment response induces changes in the directed functional connectivity of the anterior insula. *NeuroImage: Clinical, 34*, 102964. https://doi.org/10.1016/j.nicl.2022.102963

Liberati, A. S., & Perrotta, G. (2024). Neuroanatomical and functional correlates in post-traumatic stress disorder: A narrative review. *Ibrain, 10*(1), 46–58. https://doi.org/10.1002/ibra.12147

Livermore, J. J. A., Klaassen, F. H., Bramson, B., Hulsman, A. M., Meijer, S. W., Held, L., Klumpers, F., de Voogd, L. D., & Roelofs, K. (2022). Approach-avoidance decisions under threat: The role of autonomic psychophysiological states. *Frontiers in Neuroscience, 15.* https://doi.org/10.3389/fnins.2021.621517

MacLean, P. D. (1988). Triune brain. In L. N. Irwin (Ed.), *Comparative neuroscience and neurobiology* (pp. 126–128). Birkhaüser.

Manzotti, A., Panisi, C., Pivotto, M., Vinciguerra, F., Benedet, M., Brazzoli, F., Zanni, S., Comassi, A., Caputo, S., Cerritellil, F., & Chiera, M. (2024). An in-depth analysis of the polyvagal theory in light of current findings in neuroscience and clinical research. *Developmental Psychobiology, 66*(2), e2240. https://doi.org/10.1002/dev.22450

Maren, S., & Holmes, A. (2016). Stress and fear extinction. *Neuropsychopharmacology, 41,* 58–79. https://doi.org/10.1038/npp.2015.180

McEwen, B. S., & Stellar, E. (1993). Stress and the individual: Mechanisms leading to disease. *Archives of Internal Medicine, 153*(18), 2093–2101. 10.1001/archinte.1993.00410180039004

McLaughlin, K., Busso, D., Duys, A., Green, J., Alves, S., Way, M., & Sheridan, M. (2014). Amygdala response to negative stimuli predicts PTSD symptom onset following a terrorist attack. *Depression and Anxiety, 31,* 834–842. https://doi.org/10.1002/da.22284

Miller-Karas, E. (2023). *Building resilience to trauma.* Taylor & Francis.

Munoz, R. T., Brady, S., & Brown, V. (2017). The psychology of resilience: A model of the relationship of locus of control to hope among survivors of intimate partner violence. *Traumatology, 23,* 102–111. https://doi.org/10.1037/trm0000102

Nicholson, A. A., Friston, K. J., Zeidman, P., Harricharan, S., McKinnon, M. C., Densmore, M., Neufeld, R. W. J., Théberge, J., Corrigan, F., Jetly, R., Spiegel, D., & Lanius, R. A. (2017). Dynamic causal modeling in PTSD and its dissociative subtype: Bottom-up versus top-down processing within fear and emotion regulation circuitry. *Human Brain Mapping, 38*(11), 5551–5561. https://doi.org/10.1002/hbm.23748

O'Connor, D. B., Thayer, J. F., & Vedhara, K. (2021). Stress and health: A review of psychobiological processes. *Annual Review of Psychology, 72,* 663–688. https://doi.org/10.1146/annurev-psych-062520-122331

Porges, S. W. (2009). The polyvagal theory: new insights into adaptive reactions of the autonomic nervous system. *Cleveland Clinic Journal of Medicine, 76*(Suppl 2), S86–S90. https://doi.org/10.3949/ccjm.76.s2.17

Porges, S. W. (2024). Polyvagal theory: The neuroscience of safety in trauma-informed practice. In J. Tucci, J. Mitchell, S. W. Porges, & E. Tronick (Eds.), *The handbook of trauma transformative practice: Emerging therapeutic frameworks for supporting individuals, families or communities impacted by abuse and violence* (pp. 51–69). Jessica Kingsley Publishers.

Porges, S. W., & Furman, S. A. (2011). The early development of the autonomic nervous system provides a neural platform for social behavior: A polyvagal perspective. *Infant and Child Development, 20,* 106–118. https://doi.org/10.1002/icd.688

Price, C. J., & Hooven, C. (2018). Interoceptive awareness skills for emotion regulation: Theory and approach of mindful awareness in body-oriented therapy (MABT). *Frontiers in Psychology, 9,* 798. https://doi.org/10.3389/fpsyg.2018.00798

Roeckner, A. R., Oliver, K. I., Lebois, L. A. M., van Rooij, S. J. H., & Stevens, J. S. (2021). Neural contributors to trauma resilience: A review of longitudinal neuroimaging studies. *Translational Psychiatry, 11,* 508. https://doi.org/10.1038/s41398-021-01633-y

Rosenthal, M. (2019). The science behind PTSD symptoms: How trauma changes the brain. *Boston Clinical Trials.* https://www.bostontrials.com/how-trauma-changes-the-brain/#!/

Ruglass, L. M., Morgan-López, A. A., Saavedra, L. M., Hien, D. A., Fitzpatrick, S., Killeen, T. K., Back, S. E., & López-Castro, T. (2020). Measurement nonequivalence of the Clinician-Administered PTSD Scale by race/ethnicity: Implications for quantifying posttraumatic stress disorder severity. *Psychological Assessment, 32*(11), 1015–1027. https://doi.org/10.1037/pas0000943

Rustøen, T., Cooper, B. A., & Miaskowski, C. (2011). A longitudinal study of the effects of a hope intervention on levels of hope and psychological distress in a community-based sample of oncology patients. *European Journal of Oncology Nursing: The Official Journal of European Oncology Nursing Society, 15*(4), 351–357. https://doi.org/10.1016/j.ejon.2010.09.001

Schauer, M., & Elbert, T. (2010). Dissociation following traumatic stress: Etiology and treatment. *Zeitschrift für Psychologie/Journal of Psychology, 218*(2), 109–127. https://doi.org/10.1027/0044-3409/1000018

Schwartz, A. (2016, October 27). *The neurobiology of trauma-Dr. Arielle Schwartz: Informed treatment for PTSD.* https://drarielleschwartz.com/the-neurobiology-of-trauma-dr-arielle-schwartz/

Signoret-Genest, J., Schukraft, N., Reis, S. L., Segebarth, D., Deisseroth, K., & Tovote, P. (2023). Integrated cardio-behavioral responses to threat define defensive states. *Nature Neuroscience, 26,* 447–457. https://doi.org/10.1038/s41593-022-01252-2

Snyder, C. R. (1994). *The psychology of hope.* The Free Press.

Southwick, S. M., Bonanno, G. A., Masten, A. S., Panter-Brick, C., & Yehuda, R. (2014). Resilience definitions, theory, and challenges: Interdisciplinary perspectives. *European Journal of Psychotraumatology, 5,* 25338. https://doi.org/10.3402/ejpt.v5.25338

Sperduti, M., Delaveau, P., Fossati, P., & Nadel, J. (2011). Different brain structures related to self- and external-agency attribution: A brief review and meta-analysis. *Brain Structure and Function, 216,* 151–157. https://doi.org/10.1007/s00429-010-0298-1

Stephens, M. A. C., & Wand, G. (2012). Stress and the HPA axis: Role of glucocorticoids in alcohol dependence. *Alcohol Research: Current Reviews, 34,* 468–483.

Steuwe, C., Daniels, J. K., Frewen, P. A., Densmore, M., Pannasch, S., Beblo, T., Reiss, J., & Lanius, R. A. (2014). Effect of direct eye contact in PTSD related to interpersonal trauma:

An fMRI study of activation of an innate alarm system. *Social Cognitive and Affective Neuroscience*, *9*(1), 88–97. https://doi.org/10.1093/scan/nss105

Sweeton, J. (2019). *Trauma treatment toolbox*. PESI Publishing.

Sweeton, J. (2022). *The traumatic stress recovery workbook*. New Harbinger Publications.

Teicher, M. H., & Samson, J. A. (2016). Annual research review: Enduring neurobiological effects of childhood abuse and neglect. *The Journal of Child Psychology and Psychiatry*, *57*(3), 241–266. https://doi.org/10.1111/jcpp.12507

Theodoratou, M., Kougiomtzis, G. A., Yotsidi, V., Sofologi, M., Katsarou, D., & Megari, K. (2023). Neuropsychological consequences of massive trauma: Implications and clinical interventions. *Medicina*, *59*(12), 2128. https://doi.org/10.3390/medicina59122128

Tolin, D. F., & Foa, E. B. (2006). Sex differences in trauma and posttraumatic stress disorder: A quantitative review of 25 years of research. *Psychological Bulletin*, *132*(6), 959–992. https://doi.org/10.1037/0033-2909.132.6.959

Uddin, L. Q., Nomi, J. S., Hébert-Seropian, B., Ghaziri, J., & Boucher, O. (2017). Structure and function of the human insula. *Journal of Clinical Neurophysiology: Official Publication of the American Electroencephalographic Society*, *34*(4), 300–306. https://doi.org/10.1097/WNP.0000000000000377

Van der Kolk, B. A., Hodgdon, H., Gapen, M., Musicaro, R., Suvak, M. K., Hamlin, E., & Spinazzola, J. (2016). A randomized controlled study of neurofeedback for chronic PTSD. *PLoS One*, *14*(4), e0215940. https://doi.org/10.1371/journal.pone.0215940

Vankar, P. (2023). *Most stressed countries worldwide in 2021–2022*. https://www.statista.com/statistics/1057961/the-most-stressed-out-populations-worldwide/

Vialou, V., Maze, I., Renthal, W., LaPlant, Q. C., Watts, E. L., Mouzon, E., Ghose, S., Tamminga, C. A., & Nestler, E. J. (2010). Serum response factor promotes resilience to chronic social stress through the induction of DeltaFosB. *The Journal of Neuroscience: The Official Journal of the Society for Neuroscience*, *30*(43), 14585–14592. https://doi.org/10.1523/JNEUROSCI.2496-10.2010

Vindevogel, S., Ager, A., Schiltz, J., Broekaert, E., & Derluyn, I. (2015). Toward a culturally sensitive conceptualization of resilience: Participatory research with war-affected communities in northern Uganda. *Transcultural Psychiatry*, *52*(3), 396–416. https://doi.org/10.1177/1363461514565852

Wang, S., Zhao, Y., Li, J., Lai, H., Qiu, C., Pan, N., & Gong, Q. (2020). Neurostructural correlates of hope: Dispositional hope mediates the impact of the SMA gray matter volume on subjective well-being in late adolescent. *Social Cognitive and Affective Neuroscience*, *15*(4), 395–404. https://doi.org/10.1093/scan/nsaa046

Watson, J. B., & Rayner, R. (1920). Conditioned emotional reactions. *Journal of Experimental Psychology*, *3*(1), 1–14. https://doi.org/10.1037/h0069608

Weis, C. N., Webb, E. K., deRoon-Cassini, T. A., & Larson, C. L. (2022). Emotion dysregulation following trauma: Shared neurocircuitry of traumatic brain injury and trauma-related psychiatric disorders. *Biological Psychiatry*, *91*(5), 470–477. https://doi.org/10.1016/j.biopsych.2021.07.023

Wolpe, J. (1961). The systematic desensitization treatment of neuroses. *The Journal of Nervous and Mental Disease*, *132*(3), 189–203.

Yehuda, R., Hoge, C. W., McFarlane, A. C., Vermetten, E., Lanius, R. A., Nievergelt, C. M., Hobfoll, S. E., Koenen, K. C., Neylan, T. C., & Hyman, S. E. (2015). Posttraumatic stress disorder. *Nature Reviews Disease Primers*, *1*, 15057. https://doi.org/10.1038/nrdp.2015.57

Zoladz, P. R., & Diamond, D. (2016). Psychosocial predator stress model of PTSD based on clinically relevant risk factors for trauma-induced psychopathology. In J. D. Bremner (Ed.), *Posttraumatic stress disorder: From neurobiology to treatment* (pp. 125–144). Wiley. https://doi.org/10.1002/9781118356142.ch6

Chapter Three
Burnout, Secondary Traumatic Stress, and Empathy

Overview

Trauma is a major concern for trauma workers because of its link to stress. Burnout is one of the most common reasons workers leave the field. Helpers can develop secondary trauma, or compassion fatigue, when they are exposed to trauma material and do not have sufficient self-efficacy, work in an unhealthy environment, have experienced prior trauma, or lack support. Chapter 3: Burnout, Secondary Traumatic Stress, and Empathy discusses the risks of burnout, compassion fatigue, secondary trauma, and vicarious traumatization when helping people with trauma, the confusion of terminology in research, the impact of crisis and trauma on mental health, the importance of self-care, and strategies for preventing and treating burnout and secondary trauma among professionals. The chapter delineates the role of empathy, types of empathy, and neurobiological pathways, showing how affective and cognitive empathy can be harmful while compassion supports resilience. The goal is to aid the trauma worker in remaining healthy by providing routes to prevention and treatment.

Trauma Work: Are You Sure You Want to Do This?

Trauma work is thrilling and frightening. Trauma workers show passion for their roles but also must cope with the effects of their work, both positive and negative. It helps if you have the requisite training to help those with heartbreaking stories. We compare this work to the sport of noodling, a popular activity in Oklahoma, where people

DOI: 10.4324/9781003463009-3

go to the muddy rivers hoping to grab the biggest catfish. But it is a messy sport. You make your way into the river, slipping and stumbling and finally covered in mud. To grab the mudcat, you thrust your hand inside its mouth and hold tight to its slick body. This sport symbolizes what happens when we work with those who have gone through dreadful situations. Our work is mucky, and a client's pain will splatter us.

Working in trauma is messy yet rewarding. Traumatology will change you, dramatically changing your understanding of the world, people, and yourself. There may be times when you wonder why you wanted to do this. Indeed, we do not want to discourage your zeal. However, understanding that caring requires personal sacrifice is crucial.

When Helping Hurts

On April 19, 1995, the nation rippled with fear as they watched television coverage of the Alfred P. Murrah Federal Building in Oklahoma City in the aftermath of an explosion. On that day, 168 people, including 19 children, died when a Ryder rental truck loaded with explosives detonated (Federal Bureau of Investigation, 2024). Rescue workers from around the country came to help, including Chaplain Victor. His job was to comfort the family members while they awaited the news. He described the scene of worried family members, all grieving as they learned about the devastation one by one. Gathered in a church building a few blocks from the site, they learned the news had not captured how widespread the damage was, affecting numerous buildings within the radius of the bombing.

The sight of rescue workers carrying small children out of the building traumatized television viewers. Rushing to help, these caring people did not know that they would experience the long-term effects of being trauma workers. A study of 181 rescue workers from Oklahoma City revealed that approximately 10% sustained injuries during this time. A third estimated they might die during the effort. The rescue workers described crawling deep into the rubble and hearing people cry for help. In a longitudinal study, 43% of the firefighters reported long-term personal issues, while 30% developed mental health conditions. In the follow-up, 13% of the participants experienced PTSD, while 63% experienced Major Depressive Disorder (MDD). Over the next 23 years, another 11% developed PTSD, and the cases of MDD quadrupled (North & McDonald, 2023). The effects of helping those during this traumatic event resulted in long-term consequences for the helpers.

In 1998, a trauma trainer traveled to Oklahoma City to conduct a debriefing for those first responders, per the request of the Federal Bureau of Investigation. Gentry et al. (1997), developed the Accelerated Recovery Program for burnout and compassion fatigue. In the training, Victor learned about compassion fatigue and how to recover. As he listened to the stories of those first responders who were present, he became overwhelmed by their pain and reminded of his own experience. Victor shared his memories of that day as one delivering news to the families gathered. Victor shook his head as he said, "I am not sure I was very helpful." The workshop leader disagreed. "You have compassion fatigue." He hesitated, then continued. "You were doing your job." Those words comforted Victor, and for the first time, he realized the tremendous burden he was carrying in working with people who experience trauma. The next question Victor asked was, "Can I continue doing this work?"

Work-Related Stress Conditions

Like Victor, some individuals aspire to assist others, which may arise from a sense of calling or purpose or the experience of being wounded. Whatever the motivation, those entering any helping field swell with pride upon receiving the training and look forward to working with hurting people to whom they can offer sage advice and hope for the future. While novices have an intellectual understanding of the risks and are cognizant of the importance of self-care, they are unaware of the incipient hazards that arise when helping people with trauma. This innocence can lead to burnout or secondary trauma, causing impairment and preventing professionals from performing their best work (Hoppe, 2023). Various researchers agree that those helping trauma victims are at risk of emotional contagion (Lakioti et al., 2020). This research suggests that hearing a shocking narrative has a profound effect. Counselors, or other helping professionals, are privy to graphic information that leaves indelible images. Removing those from one's mind is challenging, and being unaffected by them is close to impossible. In this discussion, several terms overlap: burnout, compassion fatigue, secondary trauma, and vicarious trauma (Rauvola et al., 2019). Readers need to understand that these are stress conditions related to work and are not mental health diagnoses. None of these are listed in the current *DSM-5-TR* (APA, 2022). Burnout is the one stress condition related to work listed in the *International Classification of Diseases*. However, the World Health Organization (WHO, 2021) considers burnout chronic workplace stress, not a medical condition. Some researchers state there should be a clear differentiation between these terms as they are different constructs (Rauvola et al., 2019). Further background and information help clarify these terms.

Nurture Understanding

It is common for those working with traumatized clients to be touched and even exhausted in their work with clients. You have probably noticed people you meet who are healthcare workers (HCWs), mental health professionals (MHPs), or child welfare workers (CWWs) seem burned out. Recent statistics show that these workers have symptoms of burnout or secondary trauma.

- HCWs and MHPs with Burnout symptoms = 61%
- MHPs with Secondary Traumatic Stress symptoms = 33%
- CWWs with Secondary Traumatic Stress symptoms = 50%
- HCWs with Secondary Traumatic Stress symptoms during COVID-19 = 65% (Orsi-Hunt et al., 2023; Rushforth et al., 2023; Tessitore et al., 2023)
- As you observe these workers, which symptoms are most apparent to you?
- Do they differ among these workers? If so, in what way do they differ?

Burnout

In the early 1970s, several researchers and psychologists noticed a common phenomenon among helping professionals. Freudenberger first used the term 'burned out' to describe a chronic condition that psychiatrists and other helpers experienced because of serving others. He wrote the first book on burnout, using stories from his practice and that of other professionals (Freudenberger, 1980). Ginsburg (1974) published a scientific article on the burned-out executive. Meanwhile, several researchers worked together to bring a formal definition and quantified constructs of burnout, as well as produce an instrument to measure it. The primary investigator, Maslach, was a pioneer in burnout research. Maslach's research on burnout identified three dimensions: *emotional exhaustion, cynicism*, and *lack of perceived efficacy* (Maslach & Leiter, 2016). This information became a turning point in burnout research (Heinemann & Heinemann, 2017). Emotional exhaustion is the most common feature of burnout, otherwise described as weariness, energy loss, depletion, and fatigue. Once called depersonalization, cynicism describes the negative attitude, detached concern, irritability, loss of meaning or purpose in work, and disengagement from one's work. The lack of perceived efficacy, also called reduced personal accomplishment, refers to reduced work productivity or capability, low morale, or inability to cope with work (Maslach & Leiter, 2017).

According to Maslach and Leiter (2016), burnout is a gradual process related mainly to environmental and organizational factors. The gradual nature of burnout makes it difficult to perceive. Think of the experiment of placing a frog in a cold pot of water. If you place the pot on a stove burner and turn it on, it will slowly heat. The frog will not notice. He stays in the pot and will eventually die from the heat. However, if you place the frog in a pan of hot water, he will jump out promptly. This illustration highlights the tendency for individuals to overlook burnout until it reaches a critical point.

Going further with the research, Maslach and Leiter (2017) noted that individual elements contributed less, while the work environment played a significant role in the development of burnout. The work-related factors most salient are workload, control, reward, community, fairness, and values. When the perceived workload offers little opportunity for employees to recover and regain equilibrium, the environment creates a toxic imbalance and is ripe for burnout. Likewise, burnout rates increase when employees need more control over decisions that affect their work, low autonomy, or inadequate resources to do their jobs (Maslach & Leiter, 2016). However, when an organization provides employees with sufficient recognition for their work, values their work, offers a community of support, and creates an environment of safe relationships, it decreases the risk of burnout. Finally, when employees perceive decisions as fair and just among employees, the risk of burnout remains low (Maslach & Leiter, 2016). These are important lessons, especially in community mental health settings, which require novice counselors to carry high caseloads of highly acute patients and to meet monthly quotas to retain salaried employees.

The Maslach Burnout Inventory is one of the best to measure burnout, although other instruments are available, including the Bergen Burnout Inventory (BBI; Feldt et al., 2014), the Oldenburg Burnout Inventory (OLBI; Halbesleben & Demerouti, 2005), the Shirom-Melamed Burnout Questionnaire (SMBQ; Shirom & Melamed, 2005), and the Copenhagen Burnout Inventory (CBI; Kristensen et al., 2005). These instruments vary in their characteristics. For example, the BBI measures work exhaustion, cynicism, and a sense of inadequacy, whereas the OLBI assesses exhaustion and disengagement. Similarly, the SMBQ differentiates physical, emotional, and cognitive fatigue, whereas the CBI distinguishes physical and psychological weariness (Maslach & Leiter, 2017).

One of the most noticeable differences between burnout and secondary trauma is the requirement for empathy, although some professionals use the term compassion fatigue to describe both conditions. This lack of differentiation creates confusion among researchers and those exploring solutions. For the person who experiences burnout, as described by Maslach and Leiter (2017), the solution lies in work re-engagement and reappraisal of one's work. However, recovery from secondary traumatic stress requires a different approach (Gentry, 2022). This chapter will further explain this by examining types of empathy. According to some experts (Rauvola et al., 2019), burnout does not stem from empathy, while compassion fatigue, secondary trauma, and vicarious trauma result from empathy.

Burnout is a primary concern for workers because of its link to stress. When work stress becomes chronic, gray matter in the frontal cortex may shrink while the amygdala increases in volume. During stress, there is a disconnection between the amygdala and the anterior cingulate cortex which lessens one's ability to modulate negative emotions. In addition, sleep disturbance, a common symptom of burnout, interferes with restoration. The resulting physiological changes accelerate aging, increase lipids, and increase the risk for cardiovascular disease, Type II diabetes, obesity, and autoimmune dysfunction (Bayes et al., 2021). Burnout is deleterious to one's emotional and physical health (Figure 3.1).

Compassion Fatigue

The term compassion fatigue was first used by Joinson (1992), an emergency room nurse supervisor, to describe the burnout her nurses experienced. Even today, people

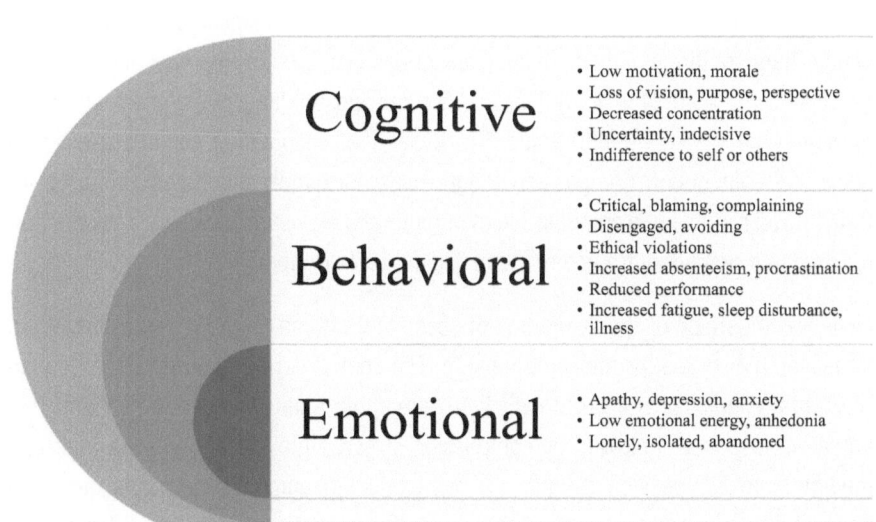

FIGURE 3.1 Symptoms of Burnout.

(Maslach & Leiter, 201M7).

in the medical field consider burnout as compassion fatigue. However, that is different from the conception of the behavioral health field. Charles Figley described compassion fatigue as he observed first responders' and therapists' experiences in responding to trauma victims. In Figley's model, compassion fatigue arises from burnout and secondary trauma, but compassion satisfaction, or one's enjoyment and reward in helping others, reduces the effects (Figley, 1995). It involves biological, physiological, and emotional symptoms that result from working with traumatized people (Pellegrini et al., 2022). Compassion fatigue can rapidly arise, but professionals can promptly treat it (Gentry, 2022). Crisis workers often experience compassion fatigue. Counselors providing disaster services in places like Hurricanes Katrina and Rita had twice the rate of compassion fatigue than counselors who did not work as first responders (Litam et al., 2021). However, compassion fatigue may also result from working with other clients.

Figley (1983) first considered compassion fatigue a burnout resulting from caring for traumatized clients. Figley recognized that some people encountered trauma because of their work with others. He noticed this with families in disasters, during wartime, and especially with workers as they responded with empathic concern to those they helped. No language or diagnosis could fully capture this experience (Figley, 1995). As he continued his work in the area, he realized burnout did not encapsulate the symptoms portrayed by these workers. During this time, the diagnosis of PTSD was under review by the American Psychiatric Association. Figley noted the critical change from the *DSM-III* to the *DSM-IV* in Criterion A1: "learning about unexpected or violent death, serious harm, or threat of death or injury experienced by a family member or other close associates" (APA, 1994, p. 424). This addition of exposure language alerted him to the missing piece in compassion fatigue. Figley identified secondary traumatic stress as a necessary component. Compassion fatigue was not simply burnout from caring for traumatized clients but a combination of burnout *and exposure* to a client's trauma that resulted in a secondary trauma reaction (Figley, 1995; Hoppe, 2023).

Figley's comparison of the symptoms of secondary trauma, burnout, and compassion stress led him to realize their relationship. The cost of caring required the following elements: exposure to a suffering client, empathic ability, empathic concern, and empathic response, followed by compassion stress. Figley recognized the path and mediators to compassion fatigue: (1) overwhelming empathic demands occurring because of prolonged exposure to the client, (2) traumatic memory recall from other client experiences, and (3) challenging or new life stressors (Figley, 2014; Figley & Ludick, 2017). Thus, when a helper cannot regulate themselves, does not have an adequate support system, experiences low compassion satisfaction, has difficulty managing traumatic memories, the work with their clients becomes intrusive, or their thoughts about the work are ruminative, and they have prolonged exposure to clients with trauma, they will develop compassion fatigue. However, if the helper has sufficient self-regulation, support, and compassion satisfaction, they will manage the residual compassion stress. Then, when experiencing prolonged exposure to clients with trauma, the degree to which they manage the traumatic memories of previous work with clients and new life stressors will determine the helper's compassion fatigue resilience (Figley, 2014; Miller & Sprang, 2017). This conceptualization is Figley's Compassion Fatigue Resilience Model, which is the concept that the energy used in empathy toward people who suffer and exposure to a client's suffering causes compassion fatigue (Figley, 2014; Figley & Ludick, 2017).

However, Figley's theory rests on the understanding that one must have empathy. Researchers hold conflicting views on this matter. While empathy may be crucial for the counseling relationship, some argue that it is unnecessary to develop compassion fatigue (Baldner & McGinley, 2016). Other studies have supported Figley's concept of a connection between empathy and compassion fatigue (Hansen et al., 2018; Zhang et al., 2020).

Our interpretation of compassion fatigue is that it results from a combination of burnout and secondary trauma. This concept means that a worker experiencing burnout is more likely to be affected by secondary trauma (Zhang et al., 2018). As a person's risk increases, burnout factors, such as systemic issues and low compassion satisfaction, are notable. Self-efficacy factors contribute to the development of compassion fatigue, including individual characteristics, such as neuroticism, personal expectations, introversion, length of time in the profession, lack of self-regulation, meaning one's aptness to moderate emotional intensity, detachment, or the ability to maintain a self-other distinction, and lack of self-care. This idea presupposes that burnout precedes secondary trauma. Burnout may enhance the risk of developing secondary trauma, but not the other way around (Ogińska-Bulik & Michalska, 2021). Exposure to trauma material causes compassion fatigue to develop in a helper, who then has an increased risk because of lower self-efficacy or burnout, resulting in compassion stress. According to Figley and Ludick's theory (2017), prolonged exposure to trauma, other life stressors, and traumatic memories, or recalling previous work with trauma material, exacerbates compassion stress and can lead to compassion fatigue. Our model of compassion fatigue incorporates Maslach's theory and

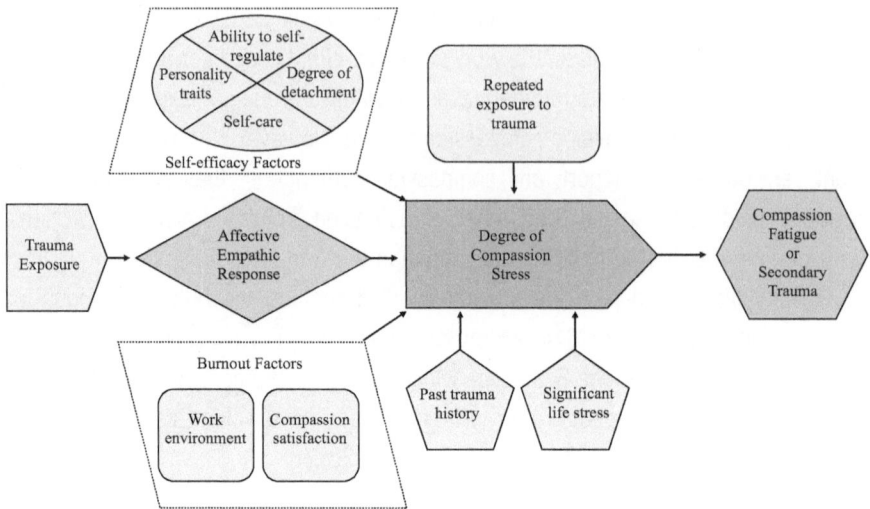

FIGURE 3.2   A Conceptualization of How Compassion Fatigue Develops.
(Hoppe, 2023).

Figley's conceptualization, recognizing the need for self-efficacy, factors that contribute to burnout, and trauma exposure, along with the helper's past trauma history and current life stress (Figure 3.2).

In identifying and quantifying symptoms in research, problems arise because the terms compassion fatigue, secondary trauma, and vicarious trauma occur interchangeably. Using these terms leads to questions about whether these are different or similar experiences. There is a growing favor to use the terms secondary trauma or vicarious trauma over the use of compassion fatigue because of this confusion, which leads to difficulties in differentiating symptoms, preventive measures, and treatment protocols.

Secondary Trauma

Secondary traumatization occurs when working with clients with traumatic memories or a PTSD diagnosis. Secondary traumatic stress is a temporary condition that is amenable to treatment (Sprang et al., 2019). People who work with traumatized clients will hear frightening details, often being exposed to the extensive violence a client experienced, which evokes psychological discomfort through an empathic response for the client.

Witnessing suffering is arduous, and therapists will sacrifice to fulfill their responsibility, sometimes at a cost to their physical and emotional health (Pellegrini et al., 2022). Secondary traumatic symptoms are like those of PTSD and result from exposure to helping someone with trauma (Cummings et al., 2021). However, the helper has not experienced the trauma themselves (Rauvola et al., 2019). The symptoms include hyperarousal, avoidance reactions, cognitive shifts in memory and perceptions, and negative mood changes (Gentry, 2022). Imagine a counselor who has prolonged exposure to traumatized clients or daily exposure to clients' traumatic material. In that case, compassion satisfaction cannot shield them from the secondary trauma symptoms they experience. Over time, helpers may develop a sense of numbness or disengagement (Figley & Ludick, 2017).

Risk factors for secondary traumatization have varied according to research trials. Most agree that the most common risk factors include exposure to traumatic material and perhaps the number of hours or time spent listening to traumatic stories (Sprang et al., 2019). It is important to emphasize that a helper can experience secondary traumatization from a single incident. At the same time, another professional who listens to multiple stories may remain unaffected by trauma. Other factors are the worker's personal trauma history and the resolution of that primary trauma. A professional with unresolved trauma is at greater risk, whereas one with resolved past trauma is at less risk (Lakioti et al., 2020).

Some studies show that years of professional experience are a risk factor, with fewer years in the field being the more significant risk (Sprang et al., 2019). The question might be whether this is because of less experience or because of placing novices in organizations that carry high caseloads with high acuity and constant exposure. According to Lakioti et al. (2020), females have a higher incidence of secondary traumatic stress than males. The incidence is higher in those who treat clients with child protective services, adult protective services, and clients with trauma. The incidence of secondary traumatic stress among mental health professionals is estimated to be around 22.7% (Aafjes-van Doorn et al., 2020). Once a therapist has secondary traumatization, what is most helpful for them? What factors should we consider for them?

Several methods exist to assess secondary traumatization. We can employ various measures to assess secondary traumatization. The most widely used is the Professional Quality of Life Scale, developed by Stamm (2010), which measures secondary traumatization, burnout, and compassion satisfaction. Another instrument, the Secondary

Traumatic Stress Scale (STSS), aligns with the diagnostic criteria of PTSD in the *DSM IV* (APA, 1994). However, neither of these scales covers all the symptoms of secondary trauma (Sprang et al., 2019).

Treatment for secondary traumatization offers various options. Self-help programs for the treatment of secondary traumatization, offered as workbooks or webinars, are popular among mental health providers. An expert panel reviewing the symptoms of secondary trauma in counselors considered the decreasing sense of efficacy, loss of empathy, and moral distress. They determined that the best approach for counselors requires both strengthening the protective factors and providing clinical treatment using evidence-based practices for PTSD (Sprang et al., 2019). As stated above, some consider secondary traumatization the same as vicarious traumatization and may prefer the use of the term. However, others believe that vicarious traumatization is different.

Vicarious Traumatization

The term vicarious traumatization is a common substitute for compassion fatigue and secondary trauma. While this is common, one should notice the subtle differences between the terms and how treatment might differ. How a helper empathizes with a traumatized client results in significant distress and possibly vicarious trauma. When this occurs with the same or multiple clients, the therapist's underlying belief systems change, transforming worldviews, views of themselves, and relational views (Kim et al., 2022). Mistrust, injustice, lack of safety, self-blame, victimization, and hopelessness dominate the helper's worldview (Padmanabhanunni & Gqomfa, 2022). Vicarious trauma can arise from working with clients on a long-term basis, such as those who have experienced sexual or violent abuse.

Preventing and protecting oneself from secondary trauma comes from compassion satisfaction or acknowledging the value of the work (Stamm, 2010). Finding purpose is another protective factor. One can continue working when one focuses on meaning and develops a career-sustaining narrative. This attenuation means moving from the role of fixing people to a position of supporting those who experience trauma. You cannot be sure of the first, "Did I successfully resolve this person's struggle?" but assured of the second, "Today I supported someone who was suffering" (Hoppe, 2023). Another protective factor is emotional self-awareness and mindfulness (Sprang et al., 2019). When a counselor stays in touch with their inner world throughout the day, even in the presence of a client, monitoring their cognitions and physiological reactions and practicing self-regulation, they increase their resilience and ability to manage the emotional overload that occurs with traumatic caseloads (Miller & Sprang, 2017). Various activities throughout the day cultivate self-awareness, or interoception, and engage individuals in mindfulness. This practice releases minor tension and keeps one fresh and focused.

Developing perceptual maturation, or the ability to reframe how one views the work, is an essential skill that aids in developing perceived self-efficacy. These skills are swiftly built with the support of peers through a self-guided program in Forward-Facing® Resilience, resulting in a competence and trauma-informed approach (Gentry, 2022). Another similar approach is the Components for Enhancing Career Experience and Reducing Trauma (CE-CERT; Miller, 2021). Both programs offer training online and in person, and individuals can purchase training materials online. The question remains how helpers can manage empathy to avoid experiencing distress. To understand this, one must explore the concepts and experiences of empathy.

Cultivate Knowledge

You have read about burnout, compassion fatigue, secondary trauma, and vicarious trauma. Describe each.

- Burnout:
- Compassion fatigue:
- Secondary trauma:
- Vicarious trauma:

In what ways are these conditions similar? How are they different?

_____

Empathy

Since some people consider empathy to contribute to the development of compassion fatigue, secondary trauma, or vicarious trauma, the discussion must include the conceptualization, process, and consideration of how to manage empathy best. Empathy can be a two-edged sword. Having empathy contributes to a successful alliance with a client or patient. According to Rogers (1975), empathy is a core condition of treatment in aiding a client. Rogers (1975) points out that high empathy is powerful and likely one of the most effective elements in client change.

Empathy is vital in the healing process. However, it can also harm the one providing it. For some helpers, empathy can lead to depression, as the helper confronts the other person's distress and induces stress in themselves (Yan et al., 2021). Understanding how this might happen requires defining empathy and its types, positive and negative.

Defining Empathy

It is natural for one person helping another to feel distress at witnessing pain. Empathy is a core condition of the helping professions (Rogers, 1957). However, one does not have to be a helper to experience empathy. Most humans express empathy. Empathy is multidimensional, referring to its multiple concepts (Baldner & McGinley, 2016). These may be either positive or negative conceptions.

Favorable terms associated with empathy include sympathy, compassion, perspective taking, empathic concern, altruism, prosocial behavior, or sensitivity to injustice. These terms differ based on several conditions, including an affective state, experiencing something like the person suffering, and being aware of one's distress versus the pain of others (Baldner & McGinley, 2016). Some describe it as putting oneself in another person's place, while others view it as a conditioned response shaped by environmental influences (Preston & de Waal, 2002). Negative aspects of empathy include mimicry, or the nonverbal display of emotion or synchronicity of facial expressions, body movements, or language; emotional contagion; affective empathy, or empathic distress, which is the adverse experience of feeling another person's grief (Baldner & McGinley, 2016):

Empathy begins early in life when the infant displays emotional mimicry, or crying, upon seeing their mother cry, despite no disturbance, hunger, or soiled diaper. Instead, mimicry results from unconsciously imitating another person's behaviors with no insight. Emotional contagion is the term used to describe the tendency to feel the same emotions as another person. Differentiating between the types is crucial before discussing the neurobiology of empathy. While subtle differences exist between terms, three primary questions can help distinguish the type of empathy.

Is the experience of empathy self-referential or self-focused, or is it other-focused?

Does the experience cause an isomorphic experience? Does the individual observing the one in pain feel distress, discomfort, or something similar that mimics the person in pain?

Is there a compulsion or drive to do something active to relieve the other person's pain? (Baldner & McGinley, 2016; Stevens & Taber, 2021; Wagaman et al., 2015)

The answers to these three questions help decipher the type of empathy one is exhibiting and may indicate a need for change to prevent secondary trauma, compassion fatigue, or vicarious traumatization.

Types of Empathy

Empathy types are controversial, but often related to terminology rather than ideological differences. In nursing, three components include an ability or action, an experience, and an expression type of empathy. The ability or action of empathy may be the underlying ability or act of providing empathy, either affectively, which is the ability to be emotionally attuned; cognitive empathy, the ability to envision another person's experiences; or perceptive empathy, the ability to distinguish the other person's state of being. Empathy can be the understanding or awareness of someone else's experience, or it can be the emotional response that it evokes. The third component of expression or communication could be a cognitive expression, stating one's understanding, or affective expression, displaying one's emotions (van Dijke et al., 2020). However, most researchers categorize empathy as affective or primary empathy, cognitive or secondary empathy, and compassion. However, some protest the use of the term cognitive empathy (Baldner & McGinley, 2016).

Affective Empathy

Affective empathy is the emotional reaction, perhaps automatic, evoked in response to another's situation. It could be a negative or positive response, meaning empathic distress or empathic concern (Echeveste et al., 2017). As a result, the helper experiences personal distress, which may lead to a higher self-absorption when they desire to help another (Kim & Han, 2018). This type of empathy is positively associated with compassion fatigue, or secondary trauma, meaning that higher empathy may contribute to compassion fatigue or secondary trauma. However, self-awareness, mindfulness, and the counselor's self-efficacy can diminish adverse effects (Zhang et al., 2020). Prolonged exposure to trauma material may cause disturbances in cognitive schemas about the safety, trust, and predictability of the world, others, or oneself. When this negative schema forms, it shatters basic life assumptions, including religious or faith principles, causes increased self-criticism and over-responsibility for problems that clients face, and diminishes the use of helpful coping resources (Padmanabhanunni & Gqomfa, 2022). The results may also affect therapeutic efficacy, loss of meaning and purpose, and alter self-identity (Litam et al., 2021). With each new exposure, the counselor or helper may develop more significant emotional distress, dissociative symptoms, poorer relational skills, or depression (Wang et al., 2014; Yan et al., 2021). Returning to the three primary questions posed by Baldner and McGinley (2016), affective empathy is primarily self-focused once a helper experiences distress, is iso-morphic, or a similar type of pain to what the other person displays, and results in an action, primarily in service to reduce the helper's distress. While this type of empathy can be harmful, there are steps one can take to mitigate the adverse effects.

Cognitive Empathy

Cognitive empathy is the intellectual attempt to understand another person's thoughts and feelings. Some refer to this as the theory of mind, the ability to take on another's perspective, or simulation, which occurs when the helper imagines the other's emotional state is their own. In contrast, the theory of mind involves attribut-ing a self-other perspective of the other person's thoughts, emotions, and behaviors (Franklin-Gillette & Shamay-Tsoory, 2021). This empathy may become exhausting for some because of the mental effort needed to gain this understanding (Echeveste et al., 2017). Cognitive empathy requires higher-order processing facilitated through the logical or thinking part of the brain (Levy & Bader, 2020). With this type of empa-thy, the focus is other-oriented or focused on the one who is suffering. The helper remains unemotional and does not feel compelled to act. The difference between affective and cognitive empathy becomes clearer in functional magnetic resonance imaging (fMRI).

Compassion

Compassion is the third type of empathy that one can distinguish. Some might call this empathic concern (Stevens & Taber, 2021). While compassion may appear to be what most consider the true form of empathy, it differs in several ways from affective and cognitive empathy. Compassion concerns others suffering and the motivation to help (Echeveste et al., 2017; Trieu et al., 2019). If a helper has compassion, they might say, "I see your pain." A person with affective or emotional empathy will say, "I feel your pain." When someone says, "I understand pain," they use cognitive empathy. With compassion, the helper focuses on the other person; the isomorphism is absent, but there is a need to act.

The Effects

It is important to delineate the types of empathy to gain insight into how compassion fatigue or secondary trauma develops. When trauma work frequently occurs over time, the empathetic helper may experience secondary trauma symptoms or vicarious traumatization (Aafjes-van Doorn et al., 2020). However, the specific type of empathy matters. Affective, or emotional empathy, activates the inferior frontal gyrus, inferior parietal lobule, anterior cingulate, and anterior insula. These brain areas manage emotion recognition, emotional contagion, and shared pain (Trieu et al., 2019). Some researchers have identified these areas with the greatest number of mirror neurons. In studies, these neurons were discovered in the mid-1990s wherein a person observing another in pain experienced a similar response to pain (Bekkali et al., 2021). If a professional helper becomes highly emotional, their autonomic nervous system will activate. The sympathetic nervous system will respond to the perceived threat, potentially disrupting the helper's cognitive skills and emotion regulation (Isobel & Angus-Leppan, 2018). The best protection against secondary trauma is an awareness of how the traumatic material is impacting one at the time of exposure (Isobel & Angus-Leppan, 2018). It is the unregulated affective response that creates distress in the helper. To combat that, one must use interoception, or the awareness of physical, verbal, or internal cues, identify the emotion and meaning, and use specific strategies during distress (Gentry, 2022; Wagaman et al., 2015).

Cognitive empathy occurs in the ventromedial and dorsomedial prefrontal cortex, anterior midcingulate cortex, and temporoparietal junction. These areas are involved in attributing mental states, theory of mind, and perspective taking (Trieu et al., 2019). While it may seem that a person will not experience distress due to cognitive empathy, it can occur. Cognitive empathy requires emotional labor, or the suppression of internal feelings that may not be socially acceptable in each situation. Instead, the helper must exhibit appropriate expressions that may be incongruent with their inner self. Doing so requires emotional energy and can become exhausting (Singh & Hassard, 2021). If affective empathy and cognitive empathy may harm the worker, what preventive techniques can the worker employ, and what treatment strategies can the professional helper use to aid?

Empathy

Tending Your Technique

This chapter mentions different types of empathy. Specific skills move one from affective or emotional empathy to compassion. The strategies needed include:

- Increasing self-efficacy (how one thinks about oneself, evaluates oneself, and one's confidence level). What activities could you suggest to a helper to increase self-efficacy?
- Increasing self-regulation (present awareness of one's physiological state, intentional monitoring of one's physiological state, and moving one's body to parasympathetic recovery). What actions or thoughts could you teach a helper to practice self-regulation?
- Maintaining healthy detachment (observing a client's pain without feeling it). What things might you suggest to a counselor to remain connected with a client but separate from them?

Many other strategies can be helpful, but practicing these skills daily will protect trauma workers from burnout, compassion fatigue, secondary trauma, and vicarious traumatization.

A Flourishing Focus

Resilience support is necessary for trauma workers and helping professionals. Whether attending an online or in-person workshop, reading materials, or practicing self-care, one cannot underestimate the importance of increasing resilience. The problem lies not in the absence of resilience but in failing to consciously utilize one's internal and external resources (Zhang et al., 2022). Everyone has some resilience. However, resilience, like a muscle, needs exercise to strengthen it.

There are several ways to prevent and treat burnout and secondary trauma. While many suggest self-care, including adequate sleep, healthy eating, regular physical activity, and time away from work, those are only helpful to a moderate degree. More than self-care is needed (Miller, 2021). The trauma worker must focus on other areas, including self-efficacy, self-compassion, and resilience. Self-efficacy is one's belief and confidence to overcome difficult circumstances (Li et al., 2019). Self-compassion employs kindness during troubling times or when failing at a task, the understanding that suffering is common to all humans, and the practice of acceptance and patience during emotional distress (Hughes et al., 2024).

To increase self-efficacy, one must increase self-regulation skills and develop a healthy empathic response, notably compassion. Low levels of mindfulness and self-efficacy are associated with compassion fatigue or secondary trauma (Kind et al., 2020). A worker's perceived self-efficacy, competence, and subjective sense of skills are important. To increase these, workers should receive professional training in trauma-informed care and using evidence-based practices. Emotion regulation, which includes changing one's thoughts about the situation's meaning and impact and expressive suppression, may help increase positive satisfaction (Singh & Hassard, 2021). Self-awareness and correcting harmful self-thoughts aid in prevention and increase self-efficacy (Zhang et al., 2020).

To increase self-compassion, the helper can find psychoeducation in self-compassion and receive compassion training. Compassion training increases activation in brain regions, allowing the professional to experience affective empathy without becoming distressed. This shift involves moving from affective empathy to compassion, which is an emotion regulation strategy (Echeveste et al., 2017).

Factors that promote and build resilience include practicing self-regulation, focusing on interpersonal strengths, using available external resources, and meaning-making, or exploring one's growth and learning from the troublesome situation. Higher resilience scores reduce the risk of burnout and a sense of care and self-care, which have a strong protective effect (Kind et al., 2020). Based on empirical studies, personal factors like resilience and engagement in mindfulness activities can lower the likelihood of experiencing secondary traumatic stress. Counselors who build resilience may effectively handle work stress, view their role as empowering clients, and boost their sense of purpose (Litam et al., 2021).

Treatment should include psychoeducation, identification of efficacious coping, trauma processing interventions, addressing avoidance, and finding meaning and purpose (Gentry, 2022; Miller, 2021). A program designed specifically for therapists, Components for Enhancing Clinician Engagement and Reducing Trauma (CE-CERT) focuses on experiential engagement, regulating rumination, creating an intentional narrative, reducing emotional labor, and parasympathetic recovery (Miller & Sprang, 2017). These practices can keep the trauma worker healthy and sustain their focus on doing the work they love.

A Flourishing Focus

Gather Self-Awareness

This activity is one way to build your resilience and self-efficacy. Follow these steps.

Step 1: Find a list of values. Read the list and choose the top 3–5 most important to you in your work life or trauma work with clients. Write them down.

Step 2: Based on these values, write a paragraph that expresses how you plan to live these values out daily. For example, if I choose authenticity, *I will strive to be truthful and authentic in my actions toward others, my clients or patients, my colleagues, and myself.*
This paragraph should be positive-focused and aim at what type of worker you aim to be.

Step 3: Shorten the paragraph to one sentence. Example: *I am here to witness suffering, to walk alongside those who suffer, and to point the way to hope and healing.*
As you read this, notice it is possible to be 100% successful daily. If I had said, "I will help everyone," I would admit that may not be possible. That can lead to discouragement and burnout and place me at risk for secondary trauma. However, the statement above is self-compassionate while being focused on what I want to do and be and achieving that every day.

Step 4: Shorten it to just a few words you can recall throughout your day. Example: *I am a witness.*

When you shorten it this way, you can remember it during the day when barriers arise and you become bored, distracted, or too emotional. Reminding myself that I am a witness helps me center myself emotionally, cognitively, and physically. I lean in and listen more closely. I move from emotional empathy to compassion. This daily practice becomes a protective force.

Chapter Summary

In this chapter, the focus is on trauma workers and the risks they face, including burnout, compassion fatigue, secondary trauma, and vicarious traumatization. The chapter highlights the risks of compassion fatigue and secondary trauma for trauma workers, emphasizing the impact of trauma exposure on mental health. It discusses the confusion of terminology in research and the role of empathy, distinguishing between affective and cognitive empathy and compassion. The chapter discusses the various types of empathy and their neurobiological pathways, underlining the potentially harmful effects of affective and cognitive empathy and the supportive nature of compassion.

Furthermore, the chapter provides strategies for preventing and treating burnout and secondary trauma among professionals, accentuating the need for self-efficacy, self-compassion, and resilience to mitigate the effects of trauma work. It addresses the importance of assessing and quantifying symptoms in research and the differences between burnout, compassion fatigue, secondary trauma, and vicarious trauma. The chapter includes the significance of increasing resilience and self-efficacy, self-regulation, and maintaining healthy detachment to protect trauma workers from burnout, compassion fatigue, secondary trauma, and vicarious traumatization. Chapter 3 provides various resources for assessment, prevention, and intervention, including coaching and training programs, assessments for burnout and secondary trauma, and tests for self-compassion and mindfulness. It also offers recommendations for resilience-building activities and treatments for trauma workers, focusing on psychoeducation, effective coping strategies, and trauma processing interventions to address avoidance and find meaning and purpose. The chapter concludes with an invitation for readers to engage in an activity to build resilience and self-efficacy by identifying their core values and developing a positive-focused statement to guide their daily work.

Chapter Review

Please respond to the following questions.

1. What are the risks faced by trauma workers?
2. What is the difference between affective, cognitive, and compassionate empathy?
3. What are the potential harmful effects of affective and cognitive empathy?
4. What strategies are mentioned for preventing and treating burnout and secondary empathy?

Chapter Summary

Key Term Assessment

Review the following terms and try to explain each concept.

- Work-related stress conditions
- Types of empathy
- Self-efficacy
- Self-compassion

Resources

The following resources may be helpful for assessment, prevention, or intervention.

- Forward-Facing® Institute, LLC, offers coaching and training in burnout and secondary trauma. Founded by J. Eric Gentry, it uses an evidence-based protocol for the prevention and treatment of work-stress-related conditions. https://forward-facing.com
- Components for Enhancing Clinician Experience and Reducing Trauma (CE-CERT) by Brian Miller can be accessed in several ways. Alyson Morgan, LCSW-S, offers a slide show explaining the model at https://panhandlebehav ioralhealthalliance.org/wp-content/uploads/2021/03/CE-CERT-ppt.pdf

    Brian Miller's book *Reducing Secondary Traumatic Stress: Skills for Sustaining a Career in the Helping Professions*, can be purchased through Routledge, online, or in major bookstores.
- Maslach Burnout Inventory™ offers several versions of the burnout inventory measuring emotional exhaustion, cynicism, and lack of efficacy. The versions include one for medical personnel, human services workers, educators, and students. https://www.mindgarden.com/117-maslach-burnout-inventory-mbi
- Professional Quality of Life Inventory offers this assessment of burnout, secondary trauma, and compassion satisfaction either in an online screening or downloadable version. https://proqol.org
- Self-Compassion Test. This online version assesses your overall self-compassion score. The individual scales measure self-judgment, isolation, and over-identification. https://self-compassion.org/self-compassion-test/j
- The Five Facet Mindfulness Questionnaire (FFMQ) is an objective test of mindfulness that measures observation, description, mindful actions, non-judgmental

inner experience, and non-reactivity. https://positivepsychology.com/five-facet-mindfulness-questionnaire-ffmq/#measure

---

References

Aafjes-van Doorn, K., Békés, V., Prout, T. A., & Hoffman, L. (2020). Psychotherapists' vicarious traumatization during the COVID-19 pandemic. *Psychological Trauma: Theory, Research, Practice, and Policy, 12*(S1), S148–S150. https://doi.org/10.1037/tra0000868

American Psychiatric Association (APA). (1994). *Diagnostic and statistical manual of mental disorders* (4th ed.). American Psychiatric Association.

American Psychiatric Association (APA). (2022). *Diagnostic and statistical manual of mental disorders fifth edition revised text (DSM-5-TR)*. American Psychiatric Association.

Baldner, C., & McGinley, J. (2016). Extracting empathy from related constructs: Historical, theoretical, and empirical support. In C. Edwards (Ed.), *Psychology of empathy: New research* (pp. 69–128). Nova Science Publishers. https://www.researchgate.net/publication/316888165_Extracting_Empathy_from_Related_Constructs_Historical_Theoretical_and_Empirical_Support

Bayes, A., Tavella, G., & Parker, G. (2021). The biology of burnout: Causes and consequences. *The World Journal of Biological Psychiatry, 22*(9), 686–698. https://doi.org/10.108 0/15622975.2021.1907713

Bekkali, S., Youssef, G. J., Donaldson, P. H., Albein-Urios, N., Hyde, C., & Enticott, P. G. (2021). Is the putative mirror neuron system associated with empathy? A systematic review and meta-analysis. *Neuropsychology Review, 31*(1), 14–57. https://doi.org/10.1007/s11065-020-09452-6

Cummings, C., Singer, J., Hisaka, R., & Benuto, L. T. (2021). Compassion satisfaction to combat work-related burnout, vicarious trauma, and secondary traumatic stress. *Journal of Interpersonal Violence, 36*(9–10), NP5304–NP5319. https://doi.org/10.1177/0886260518799502

Echeveste, U., Aliri, J., & Gorostiaga, A. (2017). Cognitive and affective components of empathy and their relationship with anxiety and depression. In C. Edwards (Ed.), *Psychology of empathy: New research* (pp. 33–50). Nova Publishers.

Federal Bureau of Investigation (FBI). (2024). *History: Oklahoma City bombing.* https://www.fbi.gov/history/famous-cases/oklahoma-city-bombing

Feldt, T., Rantanen, J., Hyvönen, K., Mäkikangas, A., Huhtala, M., Pihlajasaari, P., & Kinnunen, U. (2014). The 9-item Bergen Burnout Inventory: Factorial validity across organizations and measurements of longitudinal data. *Industrial Health, 52*(2), 102–112.

Figley, C. R. (1983). Catastrophe: An overview of family reactions. In C. R. Figley & H. I. McCubbin (Eds.), *Stress and the family: Coping with catastrophe* (Vol. II, pp. 3–20). Brunner/Mazel.

Figley, C. R. (Ed.) (1995). *Compassion fatigue: Coping with secondary traumatic stress disorder in those who treat the traumatized.* Brunner/Mazel.

Figley, C. R. (2014, April 22). A generic model of compassion fatigue resilience. *Professor Figley Polemics.* http://figley.blogspot.com/2014/04/compassion-fatigue-resilience-model.html

Figley, C. R., & Ludick, M. (2017). Secondary traumatization and compassion fatigue. In S. N. Gold (Ed.), *Handbook of trauma psychology: Foundations in knowledge* (Vol. 1, pp. 573–593). APA Books. https://doi.org/10.1037/0000019-029

Franklin-Gillette, S., & Shamay-Tsoory, S. G. (2021). An interbrain approach for under-standing empathy: The contribution of empathy to interpersonal emotion regulation. In M. Gilead, & K. N. Ochsner (Eds.), *The neural basis of mentalizing.* Springs. https://doi.org/10.1007/978-3-030-51890-5_29

Freudenberger, H. (1980). *Burnout: The high cost of high achievement.* Bantam.

Gentry, E., Baranowsky, A., & Dunning, K. (1997). Accelerated recovery program for compassion fatigue [Paper presentation]. In *Thirteenth Annual International Society for Traumatic Stress Studies Conference*, Montreal, Quebec, Canada.

Gentry, J. E. (2022). *Forward-facing® freedom: Healing the past, transforming the present, a future on purpose.* Outskirts Press.

Ginsburg, S. G. (1974). The problem of the burned-out executive. *Personnel Journal, 48,* 589–600.

Halbesleben, J. R. B., & Demerouti, E. (2005). The construct validity of an alternative measure of burnout: Investigating the English translation of the Oldenburg Burnout Inventory. *Work & Stress, 19*(3), 208–220. https://doi.org/10.1080/02678370500340728

Hansen, E. M., Eklund, J. H., Hallén, A., Bjurhager, C. S., Norrström, E., Viman, A., & Stocks, E. L. (2018). Does feeling empathy lead to compassion fatigue or compassion satisfaction? The role of time perspective. *The Journal of Psychology, 152*(8), 630–645. https://doi.org/1 0.1080/00223980.2018.1495170

Heinemann, L. V., & Heinemann, T. (2017). Burnout research: Emergence and scientific investiga-tion of a contested diagnosis. *SAGE Open, 7*(1). https://doi.org/10.1177/2158244017697154

Hoppe, K. B. (2023). A heavy happiness: A phenomenological study of compassion fatigue in Title I rural school counselors (Publication No. 30991465). [Doctoral dissertation, Liberty University]. ProQuest Dissertations & Theses Global. (2923737686).

Hughes, R. V., Hudson, K. W., Wright, E., Swoboda, S. M., Frangieh, J., & D'Aoust, R. F. (2024). Cultivating self-compassion to protect nurses from burnout and secondary traumatic stress. *Nursing for Women's Health, 28*(2), 159–167. https://doi.org/10.1016/j.nwh.2024.01.003

Isobel, S., & Angus-Leppan, G. (2018). Neuro-reciprocity and vicarious trauma in psychiatrists. *Australasian Psychiatry, 26*(4), 388–390. https://doi.org/10.1177/1039856218772223

Joinson, C. (1992). Coping with compassion fatigue. *Nursing, 22*(4), 116–120.

Kim, H., & Han, S. (2018). Does personal distress enhance empathic interaction or block it? *Personality and Individual Differences, 124,* 77–83. https://doi.org/10.1016/j.paid. 2017.12.005

Kim, J., Chesworth, B., Franchino-Olsen, H., & Macy, R. J. (2022). A scoping review of vicarious trauma interventions for service providers working with people who have experienced traumatic events. *Trauma, Violence, & Abuse, 23*(5), 1437–1460. https://doi. org/10.1177/124838021991310

Kind, N., Bürgin, D., Fegert, J. M., & Schmid, M. (2020). What protects youth residential caregivers from burning out? A longitudinal analysis of individual resilience. *International Journal of Environmental Research and Public Health, 17*(7), 2212. https://doi.org/10.3390/ ijerph17072212

Kristensen, T. S., Borritz, M., Villadsen, E., & Christensen, K. B. (2005). The Copenhagen Burnout Inventory: A new tool for the assessment of burnout. *Work & Stress, 19*(3), 192–207. https:// doi.org/10.1080/02678370500297720

Lakioti, A., Stalikas, A., & Pezirkianidis, C. (2020). The role of personal, professional, and psychological factors in therapists' resilience. *Professional Psychology: Research and Practice, 51*(6), 560–570.

Levy, J., & Bader, O. (2020). Graded empathy: A neuro-phenomenological hypothesis. *Frontiers in Psychiatry, 11,* 554848. https://doi.org/10.3389/fpsyt.2020.554848

Li, C., Lu, H., Qin, W., Li, X., Yu, J., & Fang, F. (2019). Resilience and its predictors among Chinese liver cancer patients undergoing trans arterial chemoembolization. *Cancer Nursing, 42*(5), E1–E9. https://doi.org/10.1097/NCC.0000000000000640

Litam, S. D. A., Ausloos, C. D., & Harrichand, J. J. S. (2021). Stress and resilience among professional counselors during the COVID-19 pandemic. *Journal of Counseling & Development, 99*(4), 384–395.

Maslach, C., & Leiter, M. P. (2016). Understanding the burnout experience: Recent research and its implications for psychiatry. *World Psychiatry, 15*(2), 103–111. https://doi.org/10.1002/ wps.20311

Maslach, C., & Leiter, M. P. (2017). Understanding burnout: New models. In C. L. Cooper & J. C. Quick (Eds.), *The handbook of stress and health* (pp. 36–56). John Wiley & Sons Ltd. https://doi.org/10.1002/9781118993811.ch3

Miller, B., & Sprang, G. (2017). A components-based practice and supervision model for reducing compassion fatigue by affecting clinician experience. *Traumatology, 23*(2), 153–164. https://doi.org/10.1037/trm0000058

Miller, B. C. (2021). *Reducing secondary traumatic stress: Skills for sustaining a career in the helping professions.* Routledge.

North, C., & McDonald, K. (2023). A prospective post-disaster longitudinal follow-up study of emotional and psychosocial outcomes of the Oklahoma City bombing rescue and recovery

References

workers during the first quarter century afterward. *Disaster Medicine and Public Health Preparedness*, *17*, E331. https://doi.org/10.1017/dmp.2022.296

Ogińska-Bulik, N., & Michalska, P. (2021). Psychological resilience and secondary traumatic stress in nurses working with terminally ill patients—The mediating role of job burnout. *Psychological Services*, *18*(3), 398–405. https://doi.org/10.1037/ser0000421

Orsi-Hunt, R., Harrison, C. L., Rockwell, K. E., & Barbee, A. P. (2023). Addressing secondary traumatic stress, burnout, resilience, and turnover in the child welfare workforce: Results from a 6-month, cluster-randomized control trial of Resilience Alliance. *Children and Youth Services Review*, *151*, Article 107044. https://doi.org/10.1016/j.childyouth.2023.107044

Padmanabhanunni, A., & Gqomfa, N. (2022). "The ugliness of it seeps into me": Experiences of vicarious trauma among female psychologists treating survivors of sexual assault. *International Journal of Environmental Research & Public Health*, *19*(7), 3925. https://doi.org/10.3390/ijerph19073925

Pellegrini, S., Moore, P., & Murphy, M. (2022). Secondary trauma and related concepts in psychologists: A systematic review. *Journal of Aggression, Maltreatment & Trauma*, *31*(3), 370–391.

Preston, S. D., & de Waal, F. B. M. (2002). Empathy: Its ultimate and proximate bases. *Behavioral and Brain Sciences*, *25*, 1–72. https://doi.org/10.1017/s0140525x02000018

Rauvola, R. S., Vega, D. M., & Lavigne, K. N. (2019). Compassion fatigue, secondary traumatic stress, and vicarious traumatization: A qualitative review and research agenda. *Occupational Health Science*, *3*, 297–336. https://doi.org/10.1007/s41542-019-00045-1

Rogers, C. R. (1957). *Client centered therapy*. Constable.

Rogers, C. R. (1975). Empathic: An unappreciated way of being. *The Counseling Psychologist*, *5*(2), 2–10. https://doi.org/10.1177/001100007500500202

Rushforth, A., Durk, M., Rothwell-Blake, G. A. A., Kirkman, A., Ng, F., & Kotera, Y. (2023). Self-compassion interventions to target secondary traumatic stress in healthcare workers: A systematic review. *International Journal of Environmental Research and Public Health*, *20*(12), 6109. https://doi.org/10.3390/ijerph20126109

Shirom, A., & Melamed, S. (2005). Does burnout affect physical health? A review of the evidence. In A.-S. G. Antoniou & C. L. Cooper (Eds.), *Research companion to organizational health psychology* (pp. 599–622). Edward Elgar Publishing. https://doi.org/10.4337/9781845423308.00049

Singh, J., & Hassard, J. (2021). Emotional labour, emotional regulation strategies, and secondary traumatic stress: A cross-sectional study of allied mental health professionals in the UK. *The Social Science Journal*, Advance online publication. https://doi.org/10.1080/03623319.2021.1979825

Sprang, G., Ford, J., Kerig, P., & Bride, B. (2019). Defining secondary traumatic stress and developing targeted assessments and interventions: Lessons learned from research and leading experts. *Traumatology*, *25*(2), 72–81. https://doi.org/10.1037/trm0000180

Stamm, B. H. (2010). *The concise ProQOL manual* (2nd ed.). ProQOL.org. https://www. illinoisworknet.com/WIOA/Resources/Documents/The-Concise-ProQOL-Manual.pdf

Stevens, F., & Taber, K. (2021). The neuroscience of empathy and compassion in prosocial behavior. *Neuropsychologia, 159,* 107925. https://doi.org/10.1016/j.neuropsychologia.2021.107925

Tessitore, F., Caffieri, A., Parola, A., Cozzolino, M., & Margherita, G. (2023). The role of emotion regulation as a potential mediator between secondary traumatic stress, burnout, and compassion satisfaction in professionals working in the forced migration field. *International Journal of Environmental Research and Public Health, 20*(3), 2266. https://doi.org/10.3390/ ijerph20032266

Trieu, M., Foster, A. E., Yaseen, Z. S., Beaubian, C., & Calati, R. (2019). Neurobiology of empathy. In A. E. Foster & Z. S. Yaseen (Eds.), *Teaching empathy in healthcare.* Springer. https:// doi.org/10.1007/978-3-030-29876-0_2

van Dijke, J., van Nistelrooij, I., & Duyndam, J. (2020). Towards a relational conceptualization of empathy. *Nursing Philosophy, 21*(3), e12297. https://doi.org/10.1111/nup.12297

Wagaman, M. A., Geiger, J. M., Shockley, C., & Segal, E. A. (2015). The role of empathy in burnout, compassion satisfaction, and secondary traumatic stress among social workers. *Social Work, 60*(3), 201–209. https://doi.org/10.1093/sw/swv014

Wang, D. C., Strosky, D., & Fletes, A. (2014). Secondary and vicarious trauma: Implications for faith and clinical practice [pdf file]. *Journal of Psychology and Christianity, 33*(3), 281–286.

World Health Organization (WHO). (2021). *International classification of diseases and related health problems* (11th ed.). https://icd.who.int/en/

Yan, Z., Zeng, X., Su, J., & Zhang, X. (2021). The dark side of empathy: Meta-analysis evidence of the relationship between empathy and depression. *PsyCh Journal, 10*(5), 794–804. https://doi.org/10.1002/pchj.482

Zhang, J., Wang, X., Xu, T., Li, J., Li, H., Wu, Y., Li, Y., Chen, Y., & Zhang, J.-P. (2022). The effect of resilience and self-efficacy on nurses' compassion fatigue: A cross-sectional study. *Journal of Advanced Nursing, 78,* 2030–2041. https://doi.org/10.1111/jan.15113

Zhang, L., Ren, Z., Jiang, G., Hazer-Rau, D., Zhao, C., Shi, C., Lai, L., & Yan, Y. (2020). Self-oriented empathy and compassion fatigue: The serial mediation of dispositional mindfulness and counselor's self-efficacy. *Frontiers in Psychology, 11,* 613908. https://doi.org/10.3389/ fpsyg.2020.613908

Zhang, Y.-Y., Zhang, C., Han, X.-R., Li, W., & Wang, Y.-L. (2018). Determinants of compassion satisfaction, compassion fatigue and burn out in nursing: A correlative meta-analysis. *Medicine, 97*(26), 1–7. https://doi.org/10.1097/MD.0000000000011086

References

Chapter Four
Assessment

Overview

Trauma assessments are necessary to determine the presence of any trauma experience, and specific tools are available to assess types of traumas, such as PTSD screening for symptoms, adverse childhood experiences, intimate partner violence screening, suicide screening, risky behaviors, dissociative behaviors, trauma, and abuse, and forensic screening. To adhere to best practices, care providers should inquire about specific trauma experiences when assisting individuals, couples, or families. In addition, care providers need to ask specific questions about trauma experiences. Within Chapter 4: Assessment, the reader will explore the importance of assessment and assessment methods in adults, children, adolescents, and military personnel. This chapter offers recommendations for assessment instruments and a salutogenic approach.

Where We Begin

In teaching counseling students and supervising licensure candidates, we notice client cases that increase the novice's fears and lack of confidence. Those are cases where trauma is a contributing factor during a crisis or when a client self-harms or becomes suicidal. After sharing their anxiety, these students and candidates usually ask a similar question, "Where do I begin?" Even seasoned clinicians may experience disorientation in these types of cases. We draw attention to the basic information used in other situations to solidify what they have already learned.

DOI: 10.4324/9781003463009-4

- Begin with attentive listening.
- Move to assessment.
- Determine which diagnosis is the best fit.
- Use an evidence-based approach to develop a treatment plan.

Using trauma-informed approaches, the helper focuses on four principles: acknowledging the person might have experienced trauma; recognizing trauma and traumatic symptoms; integrating the helper's knowledge of trauma during assessment; and seeking to resist re-traumatization (Howard et al., 2024). As you work with individuals, you might ask yourself questions such as, "What level of awareness do I have about trauma? Is this person's current experience related to trauma?" During your time with the client, note any observations of their behaviors, words, or trauma-related symptoms. Using your experience and knowledge of trauma, how does this change the assessment process? In what ways are you providing safety or honoring a client's autonomy? What efforts do you take to ensure a client trusts you or your organization? Are you providing the client with comprehensive information? How are you empowering the client and supporting their involvement in the assessment? Preventing re-traumatization occurs when you cautiously encourage clients to wait before sharing their entire story. Instead, focus on teaching them grounding skills such as deep breathing and staying present in the moment by naming objects they can see, hear, and touch (Menschner & Maul, 2016).

You may doubt your depth of knowledge and experience, which can create reservations about your ability to help another person. It is essential to realize that education and practice take time to develop. Instead, focus on the common factors that help most people. Developing a safe relationship may be the most impactful thing you can do. Most trauma or crisis counseling has similar healing components: the therapeutic relationship, self-regulation, relaxation, exposure or narrative approaches, and cognitive restructuring (Gentry et al., 2017).

To follow the recommended guidelines, care providers should ask about specific experiences with trauma when helping individuals, couples, or families. The first step in helping someone with trauma is asking, "In the past, have you witnessed, been exposed to, or experienced an event that was distressing to you?" We avoid using the word trauma because a person may have wounding, but not consider it as trauma. We follow their response with the next few questions. "How recent was this event? How long did it last? What effect does it have on you?" Their emotional, behavioral, and

Where We Begin

cognitive response to these two questions may highlight the need for further explora-tion. As discussed in Chapter 1, a person may face a traumatic event that is not life-threatening. In other cases, a person may encounter a life-threatening situation but never manifest sufficient symptoms to meet the criteria for a diagnosis of Acute Stress Disorder or PTSD. This situation may be sub-threshold but interferes with life's functioning (Morgan-López et al., 2023). In studies of PTSD symptomatology, negative life events may not meet Criterion A of the PTSD diagnosis. However, the symptoms may equal those of someone whose situation does meet that criterion (Howard et al., 2024). Evidence suggests that many providers fail to ask clients about trauma, even though clients express a desire for them to probe about their traumatic experiences (Read et al., 2018). Clients perceive this lack of inquiry as diminishing how their cur-rent or past treatment affects their mental health condition (Kumar et al., 2022; Lueders et al., 2022).

One reason why helpers may not ask about trauma include the fear of re-traumatizing the person. However, patients find questions about trauma no more disturbing than other questions (Lueders et al., 2022). Other providers are reluctant to ask about trauma because of their perceived lack of training or competency. This is a reasonable concern since most counseling programs offer little training in trauma or crisis coun-seling (Henning et al., 2022; Kumar et al., 2022). Others who provide help state inad-equate experience or that trauma is not their line of specialty.

However, given that many have experienced trauma, it may be impossible to avoid treating those individuals. Finally, some clinicians state they have too little time to complete a full assessment and develop a treatment plan. Unfortunately, this is akin to offering a person aspirin for a broken leg. It can lead to inadequate and ineffective treatment, if not a misdiagnosis, or further harm (Lueders et al., 2022).

The severity of the devastation, loss experienced, and the time to return to daily functioning determine the degree to which adults are affected. Other factors include the duration of the event, the number of traumatic events, and accessibility to help during or after the trauma (SAMHSA, 2014b). People have different responses to traumatic stress. Some reactions will look as expected: fear or hypervigilance, avoid-ance of traumatic material, intrusive thoughts or memories, or cognitive changes. However, these symptoms may not be apparent. Instead, the individual may exhibit anxiety, depressive symptoms, or suicidality. Sometimes, professionals misdiagnose or mislabel people. This occurrence is common among those diagnosed with person-ality disorders, substance use issues, or other mental health disorders (SAMHSA,

2014a). Traumatic stress reactions appear in marital problems, which the helper may view as a communication issue or as family dysfunction, either as enmeshment or disengagement, unaware that traumatic stress reactions are the reason. Assessment should include direct observation, a structured interview, gathering collateral information, and a reliable screening or assessment tool (Kisiel et al., 2017).

Steps in Trauma Assessment

When assessing trauma, you must ask, "What am I looking for?" and "How does assessment help?" The answer to the first question is exploring a client's presentation, or how they appear and communicate in the session, their past and current history of trauma, life, relationships, school, and work, current symptoms, recent changes, motivation for treatment, strengths, assets, and ability to persevere. There are multiple ways to explore these factors. The answer to the second question is to identify an accurate diagnosis, develop goals and treatment objectives, and understand the unique cultural perspectives of the client (Kisiel et al., 2017). A screening tool may help determine if further assessment is needed if trauma is suspected. The Substance Abuse and Mental Health Services Administration (2014a) recommends a brief screen, suicidal assessment, history review, and current needs assessment. A thorough assessment includes using a clinical interview, direct observation, collateral information, and trauma assessment tools (U.S. Department of Veterans Affairs National Center for PTSD, 2023) (Figure 4.1).

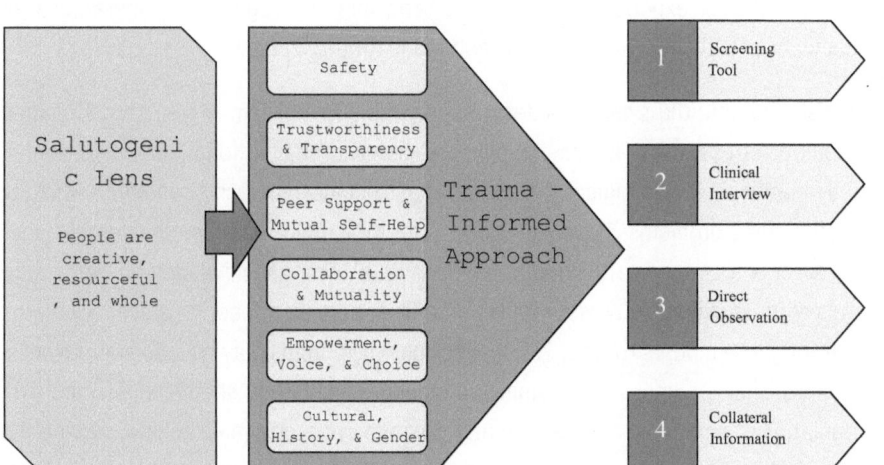

FIGURE 4.1   A Salutogenic and Trauma-Informed Framework for Assessment.

(Adapted from Kisiel et al., 2017; SAMHSA, 2014a, 2014b; National Center for PTSD, 2023).

Clinical Interview

To begin an assessment, one must conduct a thorough interview, where assessors gather needed information. Interview methods include an open interview, a semi-structured interview, and a structured interview. Through a flexible interview structure, clinicians can maintain a minimum set of questions while also having the liberty to ask extra questions or change the order and format of the prescribed questions. The flexible interview may be more conversational. However, such a relaxed interview may miss pertinent information needed. The semi-structured interview offers more structure with the questions asked in a specific order, but there is flexibility for the assessor to change some of the content. In this type of interview, the assessor asks predetermined questions. However, there is some flexibility in asking further questions during the assessment. A structured interview with predetermined questions is preferable, as it ensures you ask questions about each aspect of their life and symptomatology (Allen & Becker, 2019).

These questions should include any trauma history, exposure to trauma or violence, mental status, including mental functioning, and the presence of altered states of consciousness, such as dissociation or psychotic symptoms, which may include hallucinations, delusions, a thought disorder, or disorganized behavior. The interview should ask about self-harm, suicidal ideation, suicidal behaviors, and potential danger to others. Asking about substance use is beneficial. The interview should also explore whether the symptoms of Acute Stress Disorder or PTSD are present, including intrusive thoughts or experiences, avoidance behaviors and cognitions, hyperarousal or reactivity, and changes in cognitions and mood (Briere, 2004).

One should note the symptoms described by the client or family members. Common traumatic stress reactions may be physical, behavioral, emotional, cognitive, social, and relational. Physiological symptoms may include stomach problems, difficulty eating, sleep problems, increased heart rate, difficulty breathing, shakiness, headaches, or worsening health conditions. Behavioral symptoms include self-harm, substance abuse, impulsivity, risky behavior, and avoidance of people, places, or things that trigger reminders (Briere, 2004). Emotional symptoms may include nervousness, sadness, shock, numbness, irritability, angry outbursts, guilt, shame, significant dysregulation of emotions, or detachment. Cognitive symptoms may include viewing the world, people, or oneself differently, decreased concentration, memory loss, flashbacks, or nightmares (U.S. Department of Veterans Affairs National Center for PTSD,

2023). People who experience traumatic stress may have an increasing strain on relationships with family or co-workers. Others may struggle with functioning at home or work.

Direct Observation

Direct observation of a person's presentation is vital. When meeting with someone, what do you notice about their behaviors? Are they calm and still, or do they move around a lot, or shake? How does their voice sound? Note the tone, volume, and pitch of the person's voice. Is their speech at an average pace or too fast or slow? Focus on their mood and determine if it matches their facial expression, posture, or the story they share. Can they answer your questions, or do they take a long time to answer them, or tell you irrelevant details and never return to the question? As you observe a child or an adolescent, do they appear to be acting or talking in a way that fits their developmental age? You may notice some regression, as an elementary-aged child talks in an infantile voice, or their behaviors may be disruptive, have changed from previous functioning, or have degenerated. Children or adolescents may isolate themselves, experience sleep disturbance, or struggle in their academics.

Gain Collateral Information

Requesting additional information from those who interact with a client may be intrusive. However, a client may report symptoms that others may not know or may exhibit symptoms that others notice but of which the client is unaware. This conversation will require a release of information to consult with the client's family members, spouse, friends, physician, former therapist, or others who can provide such information. When working with children and adolescents, acquiring additional insight from teachers and other supporters is crucial. Having a fuller picture gives the clinician more insight and data to diagnose and create a plan of action.

Assessment Instruments

While a clinical interview, observation, and collateral information are vital, the assessment instrument helps by providing information about the types of traumas experienced. Specific tools exist for assessing various types of traumas, including screening for symptoms of PTSD, adverse childhood experiences (ACEs), intimate partner violence,

Where We Begin

suicide, risky behaviors, dissociative behaviors, trauma, abuse, and forensic issues. Assessment should include the type of stress reaction. Using such instruments provides another source to determine if trauma is present. Following up with a client if a screening is positive allows the client and provider to develop a plan of action addressing how these experiences affect the client's mental health. The assessment will vary based on the population, which includes adults, military personnel, adolescents, children, couples, and families with differing experiences and needs.

When assessing individuals, couples, families, or groups, maintain a trauma-informed approach that empowers individuals to leverage their strengths and plan for their needs. Always give people a choice so they have a sense of control, but work together with them, involving whoever is necessary for their care. Create safety for the person or group, recognize their physical and emotional needs, and build trust by offering respect, honor, and doing what you promise to do (Harris & Fallot, 2001). Part of offering the best possible assessment is using assessment techniques appropriate for the population: military personnel, adolescents, and children. Other populations that need special consideration are those related to culture, ethnicity, gender, people with a disability or different abilities, the elderly, and neurodiverse conditions.

Nurture Understanding

Jermaine was hospitalized for suicidal ideation. He was a 22-year-old African American male whose therapist referred for a suicide assessment. He had recently completed his college education, moved into a new apartment with a roommate, and was employed at a call center. He joined a church and became active in the college and career group. While he was excited about his new life, he began to decline. He was more than 300 miles from his adoptive parents and knew few people. He began drinking alcohol daily, but only at clubs. He thought this would be a good way to meet other people.

He soon met an attractive and successful physician. They went out on a date, but she would not return his calls or texts afterward. He tried talking with her at her apartment but could not access the locked building. One night, he called her phone at least 30 times and sent 41 text messages. At his apartment, he looked for a knife or something sharp to hurt himself. He thought life was not worth living. Fortunately, his roommate came home, found him looking, and asked Jermaine what was happening.

Jermaine broke down, and his roommate drove him to the nearest emergency room for an assessment. He was hospitalized for observation and assessment. The thera-pist requested Jermaine's permission to bring his mother, pastor, and roommate into a joint session. While hesitant and embarrassed, Jermaine agreed to this. During this meeting, the therapist learned of Jermaine's undisclosed trauma experiences, his sense of abandonment from his biological parents, and his intense desire for connec-tion with others. Jermaine heard from those present how valuable he was, how they enjoyed his presence and offers of support. That collaboration changed Jermaine's life as he realized he was not alone.

- As you reflect on this story, what thoughts do you have about Jermaine?
- How was including others in the assessment beneficial?
- What could have been the risks of including these people in the assessment?
- In what other ways could the therapist have gained the information needed to help Jermaine?

Types of Assessments

The most informative assessments include a clinical interview and an instrument to measure the trauma. However, assessments measure several things, including the types of problems and stress reactions. Once those are ascertained, reasonable steps are defined to help the person who is suffering.

Adult Assessment

Many types of assessments are available, but this chapter covers only some of those tools. The U.S. Department of Veterans Affairs National Center for PTSD, the International Society for Traumatic Stress Studies, and the American Psychological Association (APA) provide resources and assessment tools. It can be confusing when deciding which to use. This section provides some of the most common instruments in practice. Many of these are free to use and available on various websites, including the U.S. Department of Veterans Affairs National Center for PTSD. These instruments help assess adult populations. Assessments for youth and children are mentioned later in this chapter. The focus here will be on eight instruments designed to assess adult trauma, as described below.

- The *Stressful Life Events Screening Questionnaire* (SLESQ) is a self-report survey for individuals not seeking treatment. It assesses lifetime exposure to trauma through 13 questions (Goodman et al., 1998).
- The *Brief Trauma Questionnaire* (*BTQ*) is a self-report measure with ten items related to the DSM-IV criterion A1. The intention is to determine if the individual meets the first criteria of PTSD (Schnurr et al., 1999).
- The *Clinician-Administered PTSD Scale for DSM-5* (*CAPS-5*) is a companion to the LEC and provides a structured clinical interview of trauma experiences (Weathers et al., 2013).
- The *Life Events Checklist for DSM-5* (*LEC*) is a survey of 17 items meant to cover a broad spectrum of potential trauma experiences (Gray et al., 2004).
- The *Traumatic History Questionnaire* (*THQ*) has 24 items related to potentially traumatic experiences exposure (Hooper et al., 2011).
- The *Traumatic Life Events Questionnaire* (*TLFQ*) contains 21 items that measure a broad range of exposure to potential traumatic events (Kubany et al., 2000).
- The *Traumatic Stress Schedule* (*TSS*) has nine items and is primarily used as a trauma screening tool (Norris, 1990).
- The *Trauma Assessment for Adults* (*TAA*) has 12 civilian stressors related to Criterion A1 of the PTSD diagnosis in the *DSM* (Resnick et al., 1996).

These instruments assess for many types of traumas, such as assaults to self, adult sexual assault, witnessing an assault, interpersonal violence, or robbery. This measure screens for sudden or violent death, murder, or witnessing a murder, combat, or captivity. Other traumas include transportation or other accidents, natural disasters, manufactured disasters, or exposure to toxins or chemicals. Some instruments screen for abuse, childhood sexual or physical abuse, emotional abuse, or serious disease. Other traumas considered are witnessing injury, viewing dead bodies, witnessing family violence, viewing severe human suffering, or learning about trauma. Finally, traumas like a home invasion, loss of home, abandonment by a partner, abortion, and miscarriage are the focus of some assessment measures (Karstoft & Armour, 2023). The difficulty in using an assessment is choosing which one might be best for you or your client. While these overlap, some measure different traumata and differ in how they measure trauma intensity, frequency, duration, and timing (Karstoft & Armour, 2023).

Remember that assessment is a continuous process, allowing adjustments to the treatment plan or actions as needed (SAMHSA, 2014a, 2014b). In deciding how to help, a professional must consider the timing. Processing an event too soon after its occurrence may harm the individual, couple, or family. The debriefing may be helpful but should be done in a group rather than individually (Vignaud et al., 2022). Whether one diagnoses, as either a mental health provider or a medical provider, depends on various factors and is discussed in Chapter 5. The focus here is only on assessment. Using instruments designed to assess adults and separate ones to assess children and adolescents ensures the tools are developmentally appropriate.

Child and Adolescent Assessments

Children and youth are exposed to trauma frequently. In the United States, more than 65% of youth experience at least one traumatic event by the age of 16 (Lipari & Van Horn, 2017). About 21–26% of all youth under 18 have experienced at least one adverse childhood experience (ACE), and over 15% have at least two ACEs (Lyons et al., 2023). The rate of PTSD in youth is higher than in the adult population. Those children and adolescents who experience repeated sexual abuse and maltreatment or witness domestic violence are at an even higher risk of developing PTSD (Alisic et al., 2014). The prompt identification of exposure to trauma in children and adolescents is vital because of the long-term effects, such as changes in the brain architecture (De Bellis & Zisk, 2014), and potential developmental risks, as it is frequently misinterpreted as misbehavior (McLaughlin & Lambert, 2018). Age-appropriate screening tools or assessments are essential. Children and youth may be screened at school, social support agencies, or primary care facilities.

The key to assessment in children is the identification of exposure to traumatic events or other adverse childhood experiences such as neglect, caregiver issues with substance use, mental health conditions, or domestic violence. Exposure alone significantly increases the risk for PTSD or other mental health conditions (Lewis et al., 2019; McLaughlin et al., 2012). Following screening for trauma exposure, child maltreatment, family violence, or family challenges, the assessment moves to the identification of trauma symptoms, trauma reactions, suicidality, functional impairment, changes in behavior, physical changes, such as appetite or sleep disturbances, learning, or trouble in relationships. The assessor should determine if the child or adolescent has any ongoing risk of harm and report that to the state human service agency. Regulations vary

Types of Assessments

among states, so the assessor is advised to check the current legal requirements of the state where they work and where the child resides (Keeshin et al., 2020). Other helpful information in assessment is the child's or adolescent's developmental history, cultural background, history of child protective services involvement, placement, court history, current legal issues, custody, and environmental stressors (Briere & Lanktree, 2013).

The key to an effective assessment is collaboration. To ensure a comprehensive assessment, the helper must engage with the child or teen, family members, caregivers, and others who can offer valuable and continuous feedback. Building rapport with all involved will ensure that the child or adolescent receives the best care. When identifying problems, symptoms, and deficits, it is crucial to acknowledge the strengths of all individuals, the family, and the support system. Address their immediate concerns and needs. Collaborate with them to identify potential barriers or challenges. Provide additional resources or referrals for further help (Virginia Department of Social Services, 2022). When interviewing the child, Cohen et al. (2017) recommend allowing them to provide an organic, natural story. One can ask broad, open-ended questions and offer clarifying or reflective statements.

Trauma workers may need two or three sessions to complete a comprehensive assessment. During this time, one gathers information from the child or teen and family to complete assessment instruments and receive feedback from collateral sources. Assessment will be an ongoing process as new information arises. Assessment should be well-organized. This structure provides a sense of safety, ensures one can gather all needed information, summarize and integrate it, and facilitates engagement in further services needed. The challenges may include a lack of training in those assessing children and teens, a lack of knowledge about child development, a lack of time or resources, and the potential for treatment dropout (Kisiel et al., 2021).

Assessing Young Children

The assessor should focus on the problem presented in the child's context when assessing young children. Extrafamilial information through interviews with others is essential. These individuals can answer questions about the child, their reactions, changes in behavior, the quality of primary relationships, the ability of the child's caregivers to facilitate healthy growth, and the resources available (Kisiel et al., 2021). For children who are aged 0–2, trauma exposure may cause a delay or lack of development in verbal skills, memory problems, excessive crying, appetite distur-bance, or poor digestion. Children aged 3–6 may experience difficulties in learning, develop learning disabilities, misbehave, act out or imitate traumatic events, struggle to make friends, lack self-confidence, or have physical problems. The focus of assessment should be on the child's and caregivers' reactions, changes in behavior, environmental resources, attachment relationships, and the ability of the caregivers to provide healthy social, emotional, psychological, and cognitive development (Kisiel et al., 2021).

Assessment should include interviews with the child, caretakers, and other profes-sionals involved in the child's life, such as teachers, nurses, or physicians. Various instruments exist for assessing trauma in children, including:

- *Acute Stress Checklist for Children* (*ASC-Kids*) is a brief self-report measure of acute stress for children aged 8–12. It has 29 items and uses ASD diagnostic criteria. A briefer version is available (Kassam-Adams & Marsac, 2016).
- *Child and Adolescent Trauma Screen* (*CATS*) is a screening tool for trauma his-tory and PTSD symptoms in youth aged 3–18. This instrument is used during an interview (Sachser et al., 2017).
- *Child Behavior Checklist* (*CBCL*) for ages 1.5–5 (Achenbach & Rescorla, 2001).
- *Childhood Attachment and Relational Trauma Screen* (*CARTS*; Frewen et al., 2013).
- *Posttraumatic Stress Disorder Semi-Structured Interview and Observation Record* for children aged 0–4 (Scheeringa & Zeanah, 1994).
- *Posttraumatic Symptom Inventory for Children* (*PT-SIC*) aged 4–8 (Eisen, 1997).

In assessing young children, consideration regarding possible developmental delays in motor skills, speech or language delays, and sensory processing delays is neces-sary. If one is unfamiliar with assessing these delays, working with a trained profes-sional who can identify these is important. It is also vital to consider cultural and ethnic differences in assessing anyone with trauma. For example, White children tend to have high depression and anxiety, while African American children have more behavioral problems (Johnson et al., 2023).

Cultivate Knowledge

Mary and Don bring their 6-year-old, Alex, in for an assessment. They are concerned about abuse from a preschool teacher. One day, Alex came home complaining that the teacher had hurt him. Alex had a red mark on his arm but no bruises. Due to the teacher's mistreatment, Alex feared returning to school and frequently voiced his objections. Alex's behaviors changed. He started crying frequently, became irritable, and began hitting his younger brother. He was disinterested in learning and distracted. Mary and Don are investigating their legal options but want to ensure Alex will be fine.

This is your case now. Answer the following questions:

- What information do you need to know to assess Alex?
- What assessment instrument would you choose to use?
- Who should help in the assessment? Which professionals should be involved?

Assessing Children 8–12 and Adolescents

During mid-childhood, trauma exposure may include physical, sexual, or psychological abuse, natural disasters, family violence, loss or abandonment, substance use of a caregiver or self, serious accidents, severe or chronic illness, or military-related stress (Kisiel et al., 2021). Determining risk and protective factors are part of the assessment. What is the severity of the event? How close was the event to the child? How did the child's caregivers react? Is there a history of other trauma in the child's life, and what environmental factors contribute to trauma? Interviewing both caregivers and children can provide the answer to these.

- The *Acute Stress Checklist for Children* (*ASC-Kids*) is a brief self-report measure of acute stress for children aged 8–12. It has 29 items and uses Acute Stress Disorder diagnostic criteria. A briefer version is available (Kassam-Adams & Marsac, 2016).
- The *Child and Adolescent Trauma Screen* (*CATS*) is a screening tool for trauma history and PTSD symptoms in youth aged 3–18 (Sachser et al., 2017).
- The *Child Trauma Screen* (*CTS*) is a 10-item survey for children aged 6–17 and can be used by any adult care provider. It is free to use (Lang & Connell, 2017).

The above instruments will also work for young people that are aged between 12 and 17. Despite the temptation to assess the adolescent alone, it is always wise to interview a caring adult with a relationship with the youth to prevent bias. While the assessments mentioned are a place to start, many other instruments are available. Assessing a child's resilience is possible using the Strengths and Difficulties

Questionnaire, the Rosenberg Self-Esteem Scale, and the Child and Youth Resilience Measure (Rosenberg, 1979; Ungar & Liebenberg, 2005).

Assessment of Military Personnel

Military personnel, including family members, should receive special consideration during assessment. Specific traumata related to military personnel occur in six types: life-threat to self, life-threat to others, traumatic loss, exposure to violence aftermath, moral injury to self, and moral injury to others (Peterson et al., 2021). Other types of traumas include multiple deployments, adjustment to civilian life, and marital distress due to military service. The U.S. Department of Veterans Affairs National Center for PTSD recommends several assessments:

- *Primary Care PTSD Screen for DSM-5* (*P-PTSD-5*), which is a 5-item assessment tool for PTSD (Prins et al., 2016).
- The *SPAN*, whose acronym refers to the four symptoms assessed: startle, physical upset by reminders, anger, and numbness, is a four-item screening tool (Davidson, 2002).
- The *Short Post-Traumatic Stress Disorder Rating Interview* (*SPRINT*) is a 5-item self-report measure that assesses intrusion, avoidance, numbing, arousal, somatization, stress vulnerability, and functional impairment in social and vocational settings (Davidson & Colket, 1997).
- *Trauma Screening Questionnaire* (*TSQ*), a 10-item screen for all types of traumatic stress (Brewin, 2005).

In addition, one should assess military personnel for moral injury. Shay (2002) originally conceived moral injury as a betrayal by someone in authority in a high-stakes situation. Moral injury refers to psychological or spiritual injury received in response to an event wherein a person acted against or did not act which opposed their moral convictions or belief system, or was perceived by someone in authority as an act against a moral system (Phelps et al., 2022). The symptoms include guilt, shame, anger, disgust, negative self-appraisal, loss of trust, and loss of a spiritual belief system (Phelps et al., 2022). Several examples of potential morally injurious events include those involving a betrayal of one's value system, excessive violence, such as acts of revenge, or violence within ranks, such as military sexual trauma (King et al., 2023). Determining whether military personnel or a veteran have moral injury has

Types of Assessments

implications for treatment. While veterans may receive PTSD treatment, they may continue to have PTSD symptoms. This may be because interventions for PTSD do not address the symptoms of moral injury (Maguen & Burkman, 2013; Smigelsky et al., 2022). If the treatment for PTSD requires meaning-making, and someone with moral injury struggles with this process, then repair of the meaning-making capacity must occur (Kopacz et al., 2019). Assessment should explore the existence of moral injury for efficacious treatment.

Quality instruments exist to assess moral distress and injury in healthcare and military personnel. Specific self-report measures address moral distress, while others concentrate on moral injury. The scale for moral distress identifies specific distress that arises when one is exposed to scenarios and is usually related to burnout and work functioning. The instruments that measure moral injury address a broader range of behavioral and mental health concerns (Houle et al., 2024). Of the many that exist, some receive a recommendation or provisional recommendation. With high psychometric outcomes, there is a leading recommendation for the *Moral Injury Outcome Scale* (*MIOS*; Litz et al., 2022). The scale has broad coverage, distinguishes exposure from outcomes, and determines a specific index event and time frame. The instrument also screens for Criterion A and functional impairment related to moral injury (Houle et al., 2024).

There is a provisional recommendation for the *Moral Outcomes of Relationship Aggression Scale* (*MORALS*; Taverna & Marshall, 2023), the Brief Moral Injury Screen-Nieuwsma (BMIS-N; Nieuwsma et al., 2021), the *Expression of Moral Injury Scale-Military Version* (*EMIS-M*; Currier et al., 2018), and the *Moral Injury and Distress Scale* (*MIDS*; Norman et al., 2024) for military personnel (Houle et al., 2024).

Tending Your Technique

Tom was deployed three times during Operation Iraqi Freedom (OIF) and Operation Enduring Freedom (OEF). He enlisted at age 18 after graduating high school. Tom's service was typical, as he witnessed the devastation during his deployments. Eventually, Tom became a squad leader, responsible for nine other men in his company. Before his last deployment, his wife became pregnant with their third child. Much to his wife's displeasure, he had missed the birth of the first two children. Due to complications, Tom's wife was scheduled for a cesarean section. Tom requested leave to be home for the surgery and birth of his child. While Tom was attending the birth, his squad was driving, and an IED (improvised explosive device) landed near the vehicle. The result was a large explosion, killing the entire squad. Upon hearing this, Tom felt guilt and shame. If only he had been there, this would not have happened. He may have been able to prevent it. However, Tom knew this was not true but was traumatized by the event. This is your case now. Answer the following questions:

- How would you assess Tom?
- What assessment instrument would you choose to use?
- Who should be involved in the therapy process?

Increasing Assessment Accuracy

Technology and artificial intelligence are introducing new and better ways to assess individuals, especially for PTSD. Using smartphones, social media, personal sensors, and neuroimaging will revolutionize assessment and mental health care (Othmani et al., 2023: Papini et al., 2023; Wang et al., 2024). This chapter introduces self-report measures and clinical interviews for trauma assessment. However, problems arise with each method. Self-report measures may be difficult to gather, especially in children, and are also sensitive to the responder's choices. Technologies using electroencephalograms (EEGs) combined with audio and video recordings may be more accurate in diagnosing because the results can be compared with normative and predictive PTSD responses (Othmani et al., 2023). Machine learning is quickly becoming a powerful tool for analyzing multiple data sets. It can be used to classify PTSD, identify disorder onset, select treatment, and predict outcomes (Wang et al., 2024). Even PTSD risk assessment is predictable through machine-learning analysis, including self-report measures, neurocognitive results, and biomarker variables (Papini et al., 2023). These advances in precision assessment will continue to develop and contribute to future clinical practices.

A Flourishing Focus

When we assess people, we typically look for what is wrong. While that elicits a portrait of why a person is experiencing distress, it is incomplete. We must also seek what is right or assess the strengths and resiliency in people, couples, families, and groups. Why do some people fare better than others? In his work with couples, Gottman discovered that searching for what worked well helped define the problems and interventions more precisely (Gottman & Notarius, 2000). If one did not understand what was wrong, it resulted in choosing the incorrect method of addressing the problem. The same is true of those people who experience trauma. We help people best by understanding their trauma history, current functioning level and symptoms, and strengths. Traumatic events can build resiliency, and how that occurs is essential.

The definition of resilience is elemental, as discussed in Chapter 2. A person can resist a stressor, which is exhausting and can lead to further problems. Resilience is more like bamboo, which is solid but flexible and can bend in different directions. Therefore, resiliency is more than the ability to return to normal after traumatic experiences. Posttraumatic growth goes beyond that in stating that a person does not return to the same state but grows stronger (Ruud & Hill, 2022). There are several instruments useful for providers in measuring resiliency and posttraumatic growth.

- The *Resilience Scale* (Wagnild & Young, 1993) is a 25-item measures personal competence and acceptance of self and life.
- The *Resilience Scale for Adults* (Friborg et al., 2003) is a 33-item questionnaire measuring positive self-perception, positive future perception, social competence, family cohesion, and social resources.
- The *Connor Davidson Resilience Scale* (Connor & Davidson, 2003) is a 25-item tool that measures personal competence, high standards, and tenacity.
- The *Posttraumatic Growth Inventory* (PGTI; Tedeschi & Calhoun, 1996) is a 21-item scale that includes the factors of new possibilities relating to others, personal strength, spiritual change, and appreciation for life.

Including trauma and resilience or growth assessments combined with a solid clinical interview provides a richer understanding of a person's experience.

Resilience in youth and children remains a topic of ongoing research. Starting in 2005, an international team from 11 countries began collaborating to develop a culturally sensitive measure of resilience in youth. The Child and Youth Resilience Measure was the result. The study identified global aspects of resilience, along with types of tension: access to material resources, relationships, identity, power and control, cultural adherence, social justice, and cohesion (Ungar & Liebenberg, 2005). This study highlighted the areas where youth and children show resiliency.

Posttraumatic growth has not been studied extensively in children and youth, so gaining a clear picture is complex. However, age is a consistent factor, meaning that cognitive maturity and abilities help re-interpreting traumatic events. Another important factor is positive social support. Despite limited data, researchers argue that posttraumatic growth in children and adolescents resembles that of adults (Vloet et al., 2017). Focusing on the strengths, resiliency, and how children and youth grow despite or because of traumas will bring a holistic assessment experience.

This chapter has focused on the assessment of trauma. Think about how asking questions related to resilience is part of the assessment. According to the salutogenic model, protective resources may be physical, cognitive, emotional, or due to perspectives. It also includes interpersonal relationships and support networks. Completing an assessment for resilience aids in identifying a client or patient's current strengths. Think of questions one might ask that focus on strengths, hope, and growth.

Gather Self-Awareness

Everyone has thoughts and reactions to trauma assessment:

- What have you learned about assessment from this chapter, and how does it affect you?

  Sometimes, assessment seems frightening, and care providers avoid it.

- What would help you feel more comfortable in assessing trauma?

Chapter Summary

Chapter 4 focused on the critical topic of trauma assessment. The chapter emphasizes the importance of conducting trauma assessments to identify the presence of trauma and provides specific tools for assessing different types of traumas. The assessment methods covered included PTSD screening, adverse childhood experiences, intimate partner violence screening, risky behaviors, dissociative behaviors, trauma, abuse, and forensic screening. The chapter underscored the significance of adhering to trauma-informed approaches, with a strong focus on recognizing trauma, integrating trauma knowledge during assessment, and preventing re-traumatization. Additionally, it emphasized the need for care providers to inquire about specific trauma experiences when working with individuals, couples, or families. The chapter also discussed the salutogenic approach to trauma assessment, which involves empowering individuals, involving them in planning, and focusing on their strengths.

The chapter provided a comprehensive overview of assessment methods for different populations, including adults, military personnel, adolescents, children, couples, and families. It highlighted the importance of a thorough clinical interview, direct observation, gathering collateral information, and using assessment instruments to understand trauma experiences and their impact comprehensively. Furthermore, the chapter discussed specific assessment tools for adult trauma, including the *Stressful Life Events Screening Questionnaire, Brief Trauma Questionnaire, Clinician-Administered PTSD Scale for DSM-5, Life Events Checklist for DSM-5, Traumatic History Questionnaire, Traumatic Life Events Questionnaire, Traumatic Stress Schedule*, and *Trauma Assessment for Adults*. It also addressed the assessment of trauma in children and adolescents, emphasizing the need for age-appropriate screening tools and assessing resilience and posttraumatic growth.

Moreover, the chapter offered case examples and reflective questions to cultivate self-awareness and understanding of trauma assessment. It discussed the importance of considering resilience factors and posttraumatic growth in the assessment process, highlighting specific tools such as the *Resilience Scale*, the *Resilience Scale for Adults*, the *Connor Davidson Resilience Scale*, and the *Posttraumatic Growth Inventory*. Additionally, the chapter provided resources and references for further exploration of trauma assessment and resilience measures.

Overall, the chapter was a comprehensive guide to trauma assessment, emphasizing the significance of trauma-informed approaches, specific assessment methods for different populations, and considering resilience and posttraumatic growth in the assessment process. It provided valuable insights into the complexities of trauma assessment and offered practical resources and tools for care providers in their assessment practices.

Chapter Review

Please respond to the following questions:

1. What is the importance of trauma assessment in understanding trauma?
2. What tools and methods are provided for assessing trauma? How are they different?
3. What is the role of trauma-informed approaches in assessment?
4. What resources are available for clinicians conducting trauma assessments?

Key Term Assessment

Review the following terms and try to explain each concept.

- Trauma assessment
- Clinical interview
- Self-report questionnaire

Resources

Many of the assessments mentioned in this chapter are available. These resources may be helpful.

- Child/Adolescent Trauma Assessments. The International Society for Traumatic Stress Studies provides information and links to the *Acute Stress Checklist for Children*, the *Clinician Administered PTSD Scale for DSM-5*, the *Child and Adolescent Trauma Screen*, the *Childhood Attachment and Relational Trauma Screen*, the *Child PTSD Symptom Scale for DSM-5*, *Child Trauma Screen*, the *Structured Trauma-Related Experiences & Symptoms Screener*, and the *UCLA PTSD Assessment Tools*. At this printing this resource is located at https:// istss.org/clinical-resources/child-trauma-assessments

- Adult Trauma Assessments. The International Society for Traumatic Stress Studies provides information and links to the *Clinician Administered PTSD Scale*, the *Global Psychotrauma Screen*, the *Primary Care PTSD Screen for DSM-5*, the *PTSD Checklist for DSM-5*, the *Posttraumatic Symptom Scale-Interview Version for DSM-5*, the *Posttrauma Risky Behaviors Questionnaire*, the *Structured Trauma-Related Experiences & Symptoms Screen*, and the *Trauma-Related Cognitions Scale*. At this printing this resource is located at https://istss.org/clinical-resources/adult-trauma-assessments

- The Substance Abuse and Mental Health Services Administration (SAMHSA) offers a resource entitled *Family Trauma Assessment: Tips for Clinicians*. This resource focuses on assessing families who have experienced a traumatic event and best practices in family assessment. This resource is located at https:// www.samhsa.gov/resource/dbhis/family-trauma-assessment-tips-clinicians.

Chapter Summary

References

Achenbach, T. M., & Rescorla, L. A. (2001). *Manual for ASEBA school age forms & profiles.* University of Vermont Research Center for Children, Youth and Families.

Alisic, E., Zalta, A. K., van Wesel, F., Larsen, S. E., Hafstad, G. S., Hassanpour, K., & Smid, G. E. (2014). Rates of post-traumatic stress disorder in trauma-exposed children and adolescents: Meta-analysis. *The British Journal of Psychiatry: The Journal of Mental Science, 204,* 335–340. https://doi.org/10.1192/bjp.bp.113.131227

Allen, D. N., & Becker, M. L. (2019). Clinical interviewing. In G. Goldstein, D. N. Allen, & J. DeLuca (Eds.), *Handbook of psychological assessment* (4th ed., pp. 307–336). Academic Press. https://doi.org/10.1016/B978-0-12-802203-0.00010-9

Brewin, C. R. (2005). Systematic review of screening instruments for adults at risk of PTSD. *Journal of Traumatic Stress, 18,* 53–62. https://doi.org/10.1002/jts.20007

Briere, J. (2004). Diagnostic interviews. In *Psychological assessment of adult posttraumatic states: Phenomenology, diagnosis, and measurement* (2nd ed., pp. 121–135). American Psychological Association. https://doi.org/10.1037/10809-005

Briere, J., & Lanktree, C. (2013). *Integrative treatment of complex trauma for adolescents (ITCT-A) treatment guide* (2nd ed.). USC Adolescent Trauma Training Center.

Cohen, J. A., Mannarino, A. P., & Deblinger, E. (2017). *Treating trauma and traumatic grief in children and adolescents* (2nd ed.). The Guilford Press.

Connor, K. M., & Davidson, J. R. (2003). Development of a new resilience scale: The Connor-Davidson resilience scale (CD-RISC). *Depression and Anxiety, 18*(2), 76–82. https://doi.org/10.1002/da.10113

Currier, J. M., Farnsworth, J. K., Drescher, K. D., McDermott, R. C., Sims, B. M., & Albright, D. L. (2018). Development and evaluation of the expressions of moral injury scale-military version. *Clinical Psychology & Psychotherapy, 25*(3), 474–488. https://doi.org/10.1002/cpp.2170

Davidson, J. (2002). *SPAN addendum to DTS manual.* Multi-Health Systems Inc.

Davidson, J. R. T., & Colket, J. T. (1997). The eight-item treatment-outcome post-traumatic stress disorder scale: A brief measure to assess treatment outcome in post-traumatic stress disorder. *International Clinical Psychopharmacology, 12*(1), 41–45. https://doi.org/10.1097/00004850-199701000-00006

De Bellis, M. D., & Zisk, A. (2014). The biological effects of childhood trauma. *Child and Adolescent Psychiatry Clinics of North America, 23,* 185–222. https://doi.org/10.1016/j.chc.2014.01.002

Eisen, M. L. (1997). *The development and validation of a new measure of PTSD for young children.* Unpublished manuscript, California State University.

Frewen, P. A., Evans, B., Goodman, J., Halliday, A., Boylan, J., Moran, G., Reiss, J., Schore, A., & Lanius, R. A. (2013). Development of a Childhood Attachment and Relational Trauma

Screen (CARTS): A relational-socioecological framework for surveying attachment security and childhood trauma history. *European Journal of Psychotraumatology, 4,* 1–17. https://doi.org/10.3402/ejpt.v4i0.20232

Friborg, O., Hjemdal, O., Rosenvinge, J. H., & Martinussen, M. (2003). A new rating scale for adult resilience: What are the central protective resources behind healthy adjustment? *International Journal of Methods in Psychiatric Research, 12*(2), 65–76. https://doi.org/10.1002/mpr.143

Gentry, J. E., Baranowsky, A., & Rhoton, R. (2017). Trauma competency: An active ingredients approach to treating posttraumatic stress disorder. *Journal of Counseling & Development, 95,* 279–287.

Goodman, L. A., Corcoran, C., Turner, K., Yuan, N., & Green, B. L. (1998). Assessing traumatic event exposure: General issues and preliminary findings for the stressful life events screening questionnaire. *Journal of Traumatic Stress, 11*(3), 521–542. https://doi.org/10.1023/A:1024456713321

Gottman, J. M., & Notarius, C. I. (2000). Decade review: Observing marital interaction. *Journal of Marriage and Family, 62*(4), 927–947. https://doi.org/10.1111/j.1741-3737.2000.00927.x

Gray, M., Litz, B., Hsu, J., & Lombardo, T. (2004). Psychometric properties of the life events checklist. *Assessment, 11,* 330–341. https://doi.org/10.1177/1073191104269954

Harris, M., & Fallot, R. (Eds.). (2001). *Using trauma theory to design service systems.* Jossey-Bass/Wiley.

Henning, J. A., Brand, B., & Courtois, C. A. (2022). Graduate training and certification in trauma treatment for clinical practitioners. *Training and Education in Professional Psychology, 16*(4), 362–375. https://doi.org/10.1037/tep0000326

Hooper, L. M., Stockton, P., Krupnick, J. L., & Green, B. L. (2011). Development, use, and psychometric properties of the trauma history questionnaire. *Journal of Loss and Trauma, 16*(3), 258–283. https://doi.org/10.1080/15325024.2011.572035

Houle, S. A., Ein, N., Gervasio, J., Plouffe, R. A., Litz, B. T., Carleton, R. N., Hansen, K. T., Liu, J. J. W., Ashbaugh, A. R., Callaghan, W., Thompson, M. M., Easterbrook, B., Smith-MacDonald, L., Rodrigues, S., Bélanger, S. A. H., Bright, K., Lanius, R. A., Baker, C., Younger, W., Bremault-Phillips, S., Hosseiny, F., Richardson, J. D., Nazarov, A., & the Atlas Institute Moral Injury Research Community of Practice. (2024). Measuring moral distress and moral injury: A systematic review and content analysis of existing scales. *Clinical Psychology Review, 108,* 102377. https://doi.org/10.1016.j.cpr.2023.102377

Howard, J., Lorenzo-Luaces, L., Lind, C., Lakhan, P., & Rutter, L. A. (2024). Is a criterion A trauma necessary to elicit posttraumatic stress symptoms? *Journal of Psychiatric Research, 170,* 58–64. https://doi.org/10.1016/j.jpsychires.2023.12.008

Johnson, K. F., Cheng, S., Brookover, D. L., & Zyromski, B. (2023). Adverse childhood experiences as context for youth assessment and diagnosis. *Journal of Counseling & Development, 101*(2), 236–247. https://doi.org/10.1002/jcad.12460

References

Karstoft, K. I., & Armour, C. (2023). What we talk about when we talk about trauma: Content overlap and heterogeneity in the assessment of trauma exposure. *Journal of Traumatic Stress, 36*(1), 71–82. https://doi.org/10.1002/jts.22880

Kassam-Adams, N., & Marsac, M. L. (2016). Brief practical screeners in English and Spanish for acute posttraumatic stress symptoms in children. *Journal of Traumatic Stress, 29*(6), 483– 490. https://doi.org/10.1002/jts.22141

Keeshin, B., Byrne, K., Thorn, B., & Shepard, L. (2020). Screening for trauma in pediatric primary care. *Springer, 22*(11), 60. https://doi.org/10.1007/s11920-020-01183-y

King, H. A., Perry, K. R., Ferguson, S., Hicken, B. L., Jackson, G. L., Lynch, C., Woolson, S. L., Wortmann, J. H., Nieuwsma, J. A., & Parry, K. J. (2023). Identifying potentially morally injurious events from the veteran perspective: A qualitative descriptive study. *Journal of Military, Veteran and Family Health, 9*(2), 27–39. https://doi.org/10.3138/jmvfh-2022-0049

Kisiel, C., Fehrenbach, T., Conradi, L., & Weil, L. (2021). *Trauma-informed assessment with children and adolescents.* American Psychological Association.

Kisiel, C., Summersett-Ringgold, F., Weil, L. E. G., & McClelland, G. (2017). Understanding strengths in relation to complex trauma and mental health symptoms within child welfare. *Journal of Child and Family Studies, 26*, 437–451. https://doi.org/10.1007/s10826-016-0569-4

Kopacz, M. S., Lockman, J., Lusk, J., Bryan, C., Park, C. L., Sheu, S. C., & Gibson, W. C. (2019). How meaningful is meaning-making? *New Ideas in Psychology, 54*, 76–81. https://doi.org/10.1016/j.newideapsych.2019.02.001

Kubany, E. S., Leisen, M. B., Kaplan, A. S., Watson, S. B., Haynes, S. N., Owens, J. A., & Burns, K. (2000). Development and preliminary validation of a brief broad-spectrum measure of trauma exposure: The Traumatic Life Events Questionnaire. *Psychological Assessment, 12*(2), 210–224. https://doi.org/10.1037//1040-3590.12.2.210

Kumar, S. A., Brand, B. L., & Courtois, C. A. (2022). The need for trauma training: Clinicians' reactions to training on complex trauma. *Psychological Trauma: Theory, Research, Practice, and Policy, 14*(8), 1387–1394. https://doi.org/10.1037/tra0000515

Lang, J. M., & Connell, C. M. (2017). Development and validation of a brief trauma screening measure for children: The child trauma screen. *Psychological Trauma, Theory, Research, Practice, and Policy, 9*(3), 390–398. https://doi.org/10.1037/tra0000235

Lewis, S., Arseneault, L., Caspi, A., Fisher, H. L., Matthews, T., Moffitt, T. E., Odgers, C. L., Stahl, D., Teng, J. Y., & Danese, A. (2019). The epidemiology of trauma and post-traumatic stress disorder in a representative cohort of young people in England and Wales. *Lancet Psychiatry, 6*(3), 247–256. https://doi.org/10.1016/S2215-0366(19)30031-8

Lipari, R. N., & Van Horn, S. L. (2017). Children living with parents who have a substance use disorder. In *The CBHSQ report* (pp. 1–7). Substance Abuse and Mental Health Services Administration (U.S.).

Litz, B. T., Plouffe, R. A., Nazarov, A., Murphy, D., Phelps, A., Coady, A., Houle, S. A., Dell, L., Frankfurt, S., Zerach, G., & Levi-Belz, Y. (2022). Defining and assessing the syndrome of moral injury: Initial findings of the moral injury outcome scale consortium. *Frontiers in Psychiatry, 13*, 923928. https://doi.org/10.3389/fpsyt.2022.923928

Lueders, J., Sander, C., Leonhard, A., Schäfer, I., Speerforck, S., & Schomerus, G. (2022). Trauma assessment in outpatient psychotherapy and associations with psychotherapist's gender, own traumatic events, length of work experience, and theoretical orientation. *European Journal of Psychotraumatology, 13*(1), 2029043. https://doi.org/10.1080/20008198.2022.2029043

Lyons, K., Tibbits, M., Schmid, K. K., Ratnapradipa, K. L., & Watanabe-Galloway, S. (2023). Prevalence and measurement of adverse childhood experiences (ACE) among children and adolescents in the U.S.: A scoping review. *Children and Youth Services Review, 153*, 107108. https://doi.org/10.1016/j.childyouth.2023.107108

Maguen, S., & Burkman, K. (2013). Combat-related killing: Expanding evidence-based treatments for PTSD. *Cognitive and Behavioral Practice, 20*(4), 476–479. https://doi.org/10.1016/j.cbpra.2013.05.003

McLaughlin, K., Green, J., Gruber, M., Sampson, N., Zaslavsky, A., & Kessler, R. (2012). Childhood adversities and first onset of psychiatric disorder in a national sample of U.S. adolescents. *Archives of General Psychiatry, 69*(11), 1151–1160.

McLaughlin, K. A., & Lambert, H. K. (2018). Child trauma exposure and psychopathology: Mechanisms of risk and resilience. *Current Opinion in Psychology, 14*, 29–34. https://www.ncbi.nlm.nih.gov/pmc/articles/PMC5111863/

Menschner, C., & Maul, A. (2016). *Key ingredients for successful trauma-informed care implementation.* Substance Abuse and Mental Health Services Administration. https://www.samhsa.gov/sites/default/files/programs_campaigns/childrens_mental_health/atc-whitepaper-040616.pdf

Morgan-López, A. A., Saavedra, L. M., Hien, D. A., Norman, S. B., Fitzpatrick, S. S., Ye, A., Killeen, T. K., Ruglass, L. M., Blakey, S. M., & Back, S. E. (2023). Differential symptom weighting in estimating empirical threshold for underlying PTSD severity: Toward a "platinum" standard for diagnosis? *International Journal of Methods in Psychiatric Research, 32*(3), e1963. Advance Online Publication. https://doi.org/10.1002/mpr.1963

Nieuwsma, J. A., Brancu, M., Wortmann, J., Smigelsky, M. A., King, H. A., VISN 6 MIRECC Workgroup, & Meador, K. G. (2021). Screening for moral injury and comparatively evaluating moral injury measures in relation to mental illness symptomatology and diagnosis. *Clinical Psychology & Psychotherapy, 28*(1), 239–250. https://doi.org/10.1002/cpp.2503

Norman, S. B., Griffin, B. J., Pietrzak, R. H., McLean, C., Hamblen, J. L., & Maguen, S. (2024). The moral injury and distress scale: Psychometric evaluation and initial validation in three high-risk populations. *Psychological Trauma: Theory, Research, Practice and Policy, 16*(2), 280–291. https://doi.org/10.1037/tra0001533

Norris, F. H. (1990). Screening for traumatic stress: A scale for use in the general population. *Journal of Applied Social Psychology, 20*(20), 1704–1715. https://doi.org/10.1111/j.1559-1816.1990.tb01505.x

Othmani, A., Brahem, B., Haddou, Y., & Mustaqeem, K. (2023). Machine-learning-based approaches for post-traumatic stress disorder diagnosis using video and EEG sensors: A review. *IEEE Sensors Journal, 23*(20), 24135–24151. https://doi.org/10.1109/JSEN.2203.3312172

Papini, S., Norman, S. B., Campbell-Sills, L., Sun, X., He, F., Kessler, R. C., Ursano, R. J., Jain, S., & Stein, M. B. (2023). Development and validation of a machine learning prediction model of posttraumatic stress disorder after military deployment. *JAMA Network Open, 6*(6), 32321273. https://doi.org/10.1001/jamanetworkopen.2023.21273

Peterson, A. L., Niles, B. L., Young-McCaughan, S., & Keane, T. M. (2021). Assessment and treatment of combat-related posttraumatic stress disorder: Results from STRONG STAR and the consortium to alleviate PTSD. In N. V. Gornunov (Ed.), *Current topics on military medicine*. InTech Open.

Phelps, A. J., Adler, A. D., Belanger, S. A. H., Bennett, C., Cramm, H., Dell, L., Fikretoglu, D., Forbes, D., Heber, A., Hosseiny, F., Morganstein, J. C., Murphy, D., Nazarov, A., Pedlar, D., Richardson, J. D., Sadler, N., Williamson, V., Greenberg, N., & Jetly, R. (2022). Addressing moral injury in the military. *BMJ Military Health, 170*(1), 51–55. https://doi.org/10.1136/bmjmilitary-2022-002128

Prins, A., Bovin, M. J., Smolenski, D. J., Mark, B. P., Kimerling, R., Jenkins-Guarnieri, M. A., Kaloupek, D. G., Schnurr, P. P., Pless Kaiser, A., Leyva, Y. E., & Tiet, Q. Q. (2016). The primary care PTSD screen for *DSM-5* (PD-PTSD-5): Development and evaluation within a Veteran primary care sample. *Journal of General Internal Medicine, 31*, 1206–1211. https://doi.org/10.1007/s11606-016-3703-5

Read, J., Harper, D., Tucker, I., & Kennedy, A. (2018). Do mental health services identify child abuse and neglect? A systematic review. *International Journal of Mental Health Nursing, 27*(1), 7–19. https://doi.org/10.1111/inm.12369

Resnick, H. S., Falsetti, S. A., Kilpatrick, D. G., & Freedy, J. R. (1996). Assessment of rape and other civilian trauma-related PTSD: Emphasis on assessment of potentially traumatic events. In T. W. Miller (Ed.), *Theory and assessment of stressful life events* (pp. 235–271). International Universities Press, Inc.

Rosenberg, M. (1979). *Conceiving the self*. Basic Books.

Ruud, J. R. D. H., & Hill, Y. (2022). Conceptualizing and measuring psychological resilience: What can we learn from physics? *New Ideas in Psychology, 66*, 100934. https://doi.org/10.1016/j.newideapsych.2022.100934

Sachser, C., Berliner, L., Holt, T., Jensen, T. K., Jungbluth, N., Risch, E., Rosner, R., & Goldbeck, L. (2017). International development and psychometric properties of the child and adolescent trauma screen (CATS). *Journal of Affective Disorders, 210*, 189–195. https://doi.org/10.1016/j.jad.2016.12.040

Scheeringa, M. S., & Zeanah, C. H. (1994). *PTSD semi-structured interview and observation record for infants and young children.* Tulane University Health Sciences Center.

Schnurr, P., Vielhauer, M., Weathers, F., & Findler, M. (1999). *Brief trauma questionnaire (BTQ)* [Database record]. APA PsycTests. https://doi.org/10.1037/t07488-000

Shay, J. (2002). *Odysseus in America: Combat trauma and the trials of homecoming.* Scribner Press.

Smigelsky, M. A., Malott, J., Parker, R., Check, C., Rappaport, B., & Ward, S. (2022). Let's get "REAL": A collaborative group therapy for moral injury. *Journal of Health Care Chaplaincy, 28*(Suppl 1), S42–S56. https://doi.org/10.1080/08854726.2022.2032978

Substance Abuse and Mental Health Services Administration (SAMHSA). (2014a). Treatment improvement protocol (TIP) series, No. 57 (Ch. 2). In Kopstein, A., White, K. D., & Currier, C. (Eds.), *Trauma-informed care in behavioral health sciences.* Center for Substance Abuse Treatment.

Substance Abuse and Mental Health Services Administration (SAMHSA). (2014b). *SAMHSA's concept of trauma and guidance for a trauma-informed approach* [pdf file]. Substance Abuse and Mental Health Services Administration.

Taverna, E., & Marshall, A. D. (2023). Development and validation of the moral outcomes of relationship aggression scale: A measure of moral distress following intimate partner violence perpetration. *Aggressive Behavior, 49*(1), 33–48. https://doi.org/10.1002/ab.22051

Tedeschi, R. G., & Calhoun, L. G. (1996). The posttraumatic growth inventory: Measuring the positive legacy of trauma. *Journal of Traumatic Stress, 9*(3), 455–471. https://doi.org/10.1007/BF02103658

U.S. Department of Veterans Affairs National Center for PTSD (National Center for PTSD). (2023). *Common reactions after trauma.* PTSD: National Center for PTSD.

Ungar, M., & Liebenberg, L. (2005). The International resilience project: A mixed methods approach to the study of resilience across culture. In M. Ungar (Ed.), *Handbook for working with children and youth: Pathways to resilience across cultures and contexts* (pp. 211–226). SAGE.

Vignaud, P., Lavallé, L., Brunelin, J., & Prieto, N. (2022). Are psychological debriefing groups after a potential traumatic event suitable to prevent the symptoms of PTSD? *Psychiatry Research, 311,* 114503. https://doi.org/10.1016/j.psychres.2022.114503

Virginia Department of Social Services. (2022). *Conducting child and family assessment.* In Child and family services manual. Virginia Department of Social Services.

Vloet, T. D., Vloet, A., Bürger, A., & Romance, M. (2017). Post-traumatic growth in children and adolescents. *Journal of Traumatic Stress Disorders & Treatment, 6*(4). https://doi.org/10.4172/2324-8947.1000182

Wagnild, G. M., & Young, H. M. (1993). Development and psychometric evaluation of the Resilience Scale. *Journal of Nursing Measurement, 1*(2), 165–178.

References

Wang, J., Ouyang, H., Jiao, R., Zhang, H., Cheng, S., Shang, Z., Jia, Y., Wu, W., & Liu, W. (2024). Machine learning methods to discriminate posttraumatic stress disorder: A protocol of systematic review. *Digital Health*. https://doi.org/10.1177/20552076241239238

Weathers, F. W., Blake, D. D., Schnurr, P. P., Kaloupek, D. G., Marx, B. P., & Keane, T. M. (2013). *The clinician administered PTSD scale for DSM-5 (CAPS-5)*. National Center for PTSD.

Chapter Five
Diagnosing Trauma

Overview
Searching for a Diagnosis
A Flourishing Focus
Chapter Summary
References

Overview

Trauma-related stress disorders, such as acute stress disorder, posttraumatic stress disorder (PTSD), and complex posttraumatic stress disorders (C-PTSD), can be misdiagnosed as other mental health disorders, such as depression, anxiety disorders, or personality disorders. *Chapter 5: Diagnosing Trauma* reviews the history of PTSD, noting the sociopolitical influences of the diagnosis. The chapter explains Acute Stress Disorder, PTSD, and Complex PTSD, including the criteria for each. Mental health conditions, such as depressive disorders, anxiety disorders, and personality disorders, are included in the chapter as common comorbidities. The chapter discusses how these trauma-related disorders may be mistaken for other mental disorders when they may be comorbid conditions. Following this information, the author provides a salutogenic way to conceptualize treatment in case studies.

Searching for a Diagnosis

Most helping professionals intend to aid distressed people. Although some professionals train in diagnostic procedures, many fields lack specific trauma training. This text aims to ensure that all professionals working with traumatized individuals have an initial introduction and understanding of trauma diagnosis. Whether you are a mental health provider, teacher, nurse, or emergency personnel, understanding trauma effects and developing sensitivity will provide a more focused approach and offer safety to those experiencing trauma.

DOI: 10.4324/9781003463009-5

The history of trauma diagnosis is new, including posttraumatic stress disorder (Mambrol, 2018). However, for thousands of years, literature describes trauma. This history dates to at least 2027 BC, when Ur was attacked and destroyed (Ben-Ezra, 2004). Further appearances of trauma are present in art, writing, and plays. Homer's *The Iliad* speaks of the traumatic events occurring with Achilles. Shakespeare's plays, including *Hamlet* and *King Henry IV*, describe not only traumatic occurrences but also the symptoms of PTSD in various characters. Other literature depicts trauma, with examples ranging from Dinah's rape in Genesis to Shakespeare's plays (Kramer, 2016). Pinel, an 18th-century psychiatrist, wrote of Pascal's traumatic experience wherein his horses bolted, throwing the carriage into the Seine, where he came close to drowning (1797). The Greek historian Herodotus of Heraklion described traumatic reactions when writing about the history of England and France (Kucmin et al., 2016).

However, the first scientific descriptions occur in the writings of the Napoleonic Wars (Birmes et al., 2003). Some called traumatic experiences by different names, including Soldier's Heart, irritable heart syndrome, war neurosis, shell shock, and battle fatigue (Kucmin et al., 2016). Janet was the first to correlate unconscious memories with neurotic memories in his work, *L'Automatisme Psychologique*, where at least half of the case studies described the result of psychological trauma. In the 1880s, Charcot, in explaining a case of hysteria related to a woman's dissociative state to prior abuse, called it nervous shock (Micale, 1995). Charcot's work noted the connection between females suffering from hysteria and childhood sexual abuse (Mambrol, 2018). Freud included this concept of abuse in *The Aetiology of Hysteria*. Influenced by Jean-Martin Charcot, Freud focused on treating trauma memories (Mambrol, 2018). However, the social and political environment reacted against this proposal, so Freud retracted his theory. He returned to the theory in his *Introductory Letters on Psychoanalysis* (Spiers & Harrington, 2001).

Unlike other mental health disorders, the proposal of PTSD has swirled with controversy, influenced by political and sociocultural climates. Some worried that such a diagnosis would increase the number of liability claims, while others posited that traumatic reports were unreliable and possibly invalid (Kucmin et al., 2016). Several convergent social movements led by veterans, Holocaust survivors, and feminists influenced the inclusion of PTSD in the *DSM*. The trauma diagnosis first appeared in the American Psychiatric Association (APA) *DSM-III* in 1980 (APA, 1980; Friedman et al., 2021). Initially, mental health professionals viewed PTSD as a catastrophic stress occurring outside the range of typical human experience (Friedman, 2023). A recognizable stress that evoked significant distress in nearly everyone, symptoms of re-experiencing, at least one indicator of numbing or avoidance, and at least several symptoms of physiological reactions or negative cognitive shifts were used for the diagnosis in the *DSM-III* (APA, 1980). The typical symptoms or effects of war, torture, rape, or natural disasters, such as earthquakes, tornados, hurricanes, and human-made disasters, including explosions and transportation accidents, met the criteria for a calamitous event (APA, 1980). This perception ruled out painful incidences, including divorce, serious illness, and financial failure. Instead, these events were considered adjustment disorders (Friedman, 2023). The third edition of the *DSM* classified PTSD as an anxiety disorder based on the symptoms of Vietnam veterans. In the meantime, the World Health Organization (WHO) *International Classification of Disorders* (*ICD-10*) included a similar perspective (WHO, 1999).

By working with various organizations and conducting research, the *DSM-IV* expanded its definition of trauma to encompass a more comprehensive understanding (Substance Abuse and Mental Health Services Administration, 2014). In addition, the *DSM-IV* included exposure to trauma, intrusive recollections, avoidance, and hyperarousal symptoms (Friedman, 2023). The *DSM-5* reclassified PTSD as a Trauma- and Stressor-Related Disorder (Friedman, 2023). Acute Stress Disorder appeared as a diagnosis in the *DSM-IV* published in 1994 (APA, 1994). This diagnosis identified the early potential for PTSD and enabled third-party payors to support the treatment for individuals. The diagnosis sought to bridge the gap for those people having an acute reaction to trauma stress (Cardeña & Carlson, 2011).

Trauma Diagnoses

Not everyone exposed to trauma develops Acute Stress Disorder or PTSD. Some people may develop subsequent depression, anxiety, or other mental health disorders. Other individuals will have temporal symptoms that dissipate and receive no diagnosis (Cardeña & Carlson, 2011). This incidence varies depending on risk and protective factors (Schein et al., 2021). However, a basic understanding of these diagnoses helps formulate treatment planning. Acute Stress Disorder, PTSD, and Complex PTSD are further discussed and compared.

Acute Stress Disorder

Following a traumatic occurrence, a significant number of individuals undergo an initial intense stress response. Specific individuals may encounter dissociative symptoms and struggle to recall specifics of the traumatic event. At first, healthcare professionals referred to this condition as a brief reactive dissociative disorder. It involved the presence of at least one of the following symptoms: stupor, derealization, depersonalization, perceptual distortions, emotional numbing or detachment from others, psychogenic amnesia, or physiological hyperarousal. Nevertheless, the editors of the *DSM-IV*, under the leadership of the Anxiety Disorders Work Force, concluded that Acute Stress Disorder provided a more precise description of the illness (Cardeña & Carlson, 2011).

According to the *DSM-5-TR*, Acute Stress Disorder is a psychological condition that is defined by a response to a traumatic event that occurs because of direct experience, witnessing the incident in person, knowing about it happening to a close family member or acquaintance, or recurrent and intense exposure to disturbing details (APA, 2022). Media exposure is exempt from this requirement unless mandated by the workplace. To meet the criteria for diagnosis, an individual must exhibit at least nine symptoms from any of the five categories: intrusion, negative mood, dissociation, avoidance, and arousal (APA, 2022). The symptoms of Acute Stress Disorder closely resemble those of PTSD. However, unlike PTSD, Acute Stress Disorder does not involve fear-based symptoms such as engaging in risky or harmful conduct or experiencing negative thoughts (U.S. Department of Veterans Affairs, 2024a). The distinction between PTSD and Acute Stress Disorder lies in the timeframe and the occurrence of dissociative experiences, which serve as indicators for the development of PTSD (Bryant et al., 2011). The symptoms of Acute Stress Disorder manifest after experiencing a traumatic event and persist for a minimum of three days and a maximum of one month (APA, 2022).

The prevalence of Acute Stress Disorder varies, dependent on when people report their symptoms, with rates of 11.7% to 40.6% (Fanai & Khan, 2024; Geoffrion et al., 2022). The prevalence of Acute Stress Disorder depends on the type of trauma. Higher rates occur following interpersonal trauma, motor vehicle accidents, a life-threatening illness, or disasters (Geoffrion et al., 2022). Conceptualization of Acute Stress Disorder requires understanding the immediacy of symptoms and the need for stabilization. This concept means successful interventions should include psychological first-aid models or debriefing. According to the U.S. Department of Veterans Affairs (VA), addressing the initial symptoms may or may not prevent the development of PTSD, but it can be helpful for individuals (VA, 2024a).

Nurture Understanding

Donnie, a married male who was 35 years old, works at a correctional facility for young men aged 12–18. He loves his work there, but a robust youth attacked him a week ago, resulting in Donnie's neck and back being injured. As a result, he is having difficulty walking and participating in enjoyable activities. Donnie complains of intense nightmares intense arousal when driving by his former workplace, and so he avoids driving in that part of town, ignores calls from his workplace, and avoids his colleagues. He is irritable and not sleeping well and also complains of difficulty paying attention. This illustrates a recent traumatic event. Answer the following questions:

- Does Donnie have Acute Stress Disorder?
- What symptoms do you see present?
- Where would you start in helping Donnie?

Posttraumatic Stress Disorder (PTSD)

The diagnosis of PTSD continues to be controversial for several reasons. First, some might consider it a normal response to human stressors. The *DSM-5-TR* views PTSD as a distinct disorder that impairs social, relational, and other life functioning (APA, 2022). Secondly, there are individuals who do not meet at least one criterion for PTSD, and so receive a different diagnosis (Levin-Aspenson & Greene, 2024; Flory & Yehuda, 2015). Others argue that posttraumatic symptoms appear in ordinary activities, such as childbirth, surgery, or work displacement (Bryant, 2023). The challenge in diagnosing PTSD is the prevalence of those people with subthreshold symptoms or an insufficient number or severity of symptoms to meet the full criteria (Marshall et al., 2001). These individuals may receive another diagnosis with their trauma symptoms minimized; thus, appropriate care and treatment will be unlikely. While research for PTSD biomarkers has been unsuccessful in identifying PTSD, other studies using machine learning of biomedical data, including psychophysiological factors, endocrine levels, prescribed pharmacotherapy, and psychological assessments, have been successful in predicting stress severity at 12 months (Schultebraucks et al., 2021).

The *DSM-5-TR* outlines the criteria for PTSD, which involves exposure to trauma such as death, threatened death, serious injury, or sexual violence. This exposure can occur through direct experience, witnessing the event, learning about it happening to a close family member or friend, or repeated and intense exposure to distressing details of the trauma (APA, 2022). The *DSM-5-TR* does not consider exposure through media unless it is necessary for a person's job to view traumatic material. An individual must exhibit four distinct groups of symptoms: intrusive symptoms, persistent avoidance,

Searching for a Diagnosis

unfavorable alterations in thinking or mood, and significant changes in arousal and reactivity. All of these symptoms are linked to a traumatic event (APA, 2022). Examples of symptoms within the four clusters include the following:

- Intrusion symptoms manifest frequently and persistently, are involuntary, and may consist of disturbing recollections related to the traumatic event. An individual may experience nightmares or exhibit dissociative responses, such as flashbacks. During that period, the individual's response indicates that they see the trauma as still happening. These occurrences are transient yet severe and cause psychological anguish. Intrusion symptoms might manifest when internal or external stimuli are present that are reminders of the traumatic event (APA, 2022).
- Avoidance symptoms refer to deliberate actions that a person takes to evade uncomfortable memories, thoughts, or emotions. It can also refer to avoiding individuals, locations, objects, or activities that trigger unpleasant recollections, thoughts, or emotions (APA, 2022).
- Adverse cognitive and emotional changes may encompass amnesia regarding the traumatic event; persistent and magnified self-perceptions, impractical anticipations of oneself, others, or the world; distorted thoughts regarding the origin of the trauma; self-reproach, continual negative emotions like fear, shame, or guilt; anhedonia; a sense of detachment, and an incapacity to experience positive emotions (APA, 2022).
- Notable alterations in alertness and responsiveness. These symptoms can manifest as persistent irritability, sudden bursts of anger without much reason, heightened vigilance, or reduced ability to concentrate or sleep well (APA, 2022).

In order to meet the criteria, these symptoms must persist for at least one month and result in considerable distress or impairment in a person's interpersonal relationships or occupational functioning. Furthermore, the diagnostician must assess for dissociative symptoms, such as depersonalization, which refers to a persistent or recurring feeling of detachment or observing one's internal or physical experiences from an external perspective, and derealization, which involves a persistent or recurring sense of the world being unreal, dreamlike, distant, or distorted (APA, 2022). In the most recent version, *DSM-5-TR*, the only modifications made were to the A2 criteria for children aged six and below. In the case of children, the diagnosis is based on behavioral signs rather than abstract concepts (Scheeringa, 2023) (Figure 5.1).

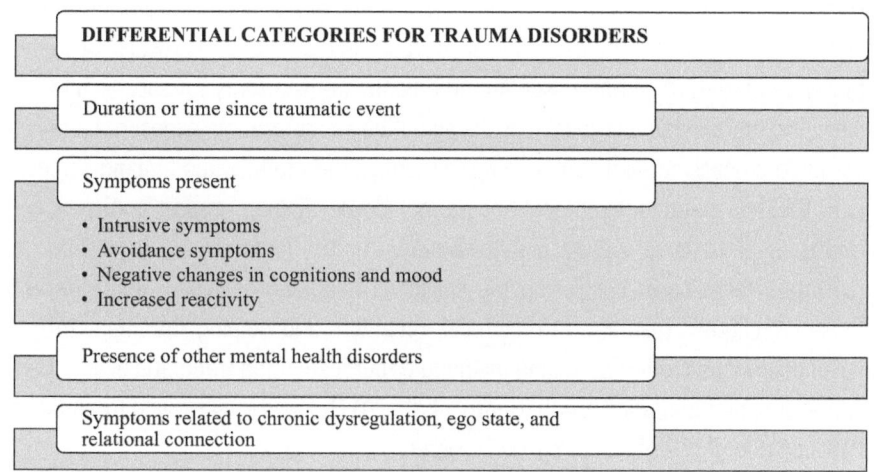

DIFFERENTIAL CATEGORIES FOR TRAUMA DISORDERS

Duration or time since traumatic event

Symptoms present

- Intrusive symptoms
- Avoidance symptoms
- Negative changes in cognitions and mood
- Increased reactivity

Presence of other mental health disorders

Symptoms related to chronic dysregulation, ego state, and relational connection

FIGURE 5.1   Differential Categories for Trauma Disorders.

To meet the diagnostic, an individual must exhibit these symptoms for over a month and experience notable distress or impairment in critical areas of their daily functioning. Furthermore, substances or medical conditions must not be the source of the symptoms (APA, 2022). The lifetime prevalence of PTSD is between 3.4% and 26.9% in the U.S. population. In military personnel, the lifetime prevalence ranges from 7.7% to 17.0% (Schein et al., 2021). Risk factors for PTSD include a dosage effect or the number of traumas a person experiences. In addition, a history of mental health symptoms, being female, job satisfaction, lack of social support, or ineffective coping strategies may predispose people to PTSD. Other risk factors include individual personality characteristics such as avoidance coping strategies, detached engagement, or impulsivity (Henninger, 2021). Early childhood factors, parental dysfunction, and a child's home life account for 12% of the variance in PTSD symptoms. Past severe stressors and the age of the first trauma are also significant, with an earlier age associated with an increased risk for PTSD (Carlson et al., 2016).

Protective factors for PTSD include individual characteristics such as cognitive flexibility, trait resilience, secure attachment, social support, adaptive coping skills, optimism, and general self-efficacy (Campodonico et al., 2021; Henninger, 2021). Sociocultural factors protect individuals and include higher IQs (intelligence quotients), higher education, family cohesion, and positive parenting (Henninger, 2021).

Searching for a Diagnosis

Understanding that PTSD arises from intrusive symptoms linked to the initial traumatic event rather than the trauma itself is crucial in the treatment process. According to Gentry et al. (2017), four essential ingredients are necessary for successful treatment: the therapeutic relationship; self-regulation and relaxation; exposure therapy or narrative processing; and cognitive restructuring. Therefore, when helping someone with PTSD, a treatment protocol should include developing rapport and trust with clients or patients; providing psychoeducation and practice in self-regulation and relaxation techniques; combining the narrative, imaginal, or in vivo exposure with those techniques, resulting in reciprocal inhibition; and helping the client to form novel approaches to life or finding meaning or purpose in the traumatic event, which will allow posttraumatic growth (Gentry et al., 2017). The diagnosis and treatment of PTSD parallel those of Acute Stress Disorder.

Cultivate Knowledge

Do you need help remembering the categories of criteria for PTSD? Try creating a mnemonic device. For example, here's one that helps us remember: After learning that elephants, which we love, are on the endangered species list, we explored more about them and why they are disappearing. That made an impression on us, so we decided to create our own mnemonic device using this information: Elephants In Africa Need Apples. Here is how these relate to trauma.

- Elephants – PTSD must include Exposure to a traumatic event.
- In – Due to the exposure, one experiences Intrusive thoughts and memories of the event, such as nightmares or flashbacks.
- Africa is where most elephants live, but some people also hope to visit and go on safari there. This part of the mnemonic symbolizes the Avoidance of people, places, and things that remind or trigger emotional reactions.
- Need – Elephants have many needs. People with PTSD need help but have difficulty asking for it due to their Negative thoughts. They may feel guilty, undeserving or develop a negative outlook.
- Apples – Elephants eat a lot of food. Typically, they eat fruits and vegetables. They can eat up to 400 pounds of food daily – a lot of apples. People with trauma have symptoms of Arousal, usually a heightened startle response or an overreaction to slight movements or commands.

While that does not cover all the criteria, it helps you remember the symptom categories. Now it's your turn to create your own mnemonic device to remember these symptom categories.

Complex PTSD and Developmental Trauma Disorder

Some people experience additional symptoms of PTSD because of repeated victimization. While the *DSM-5-TR* does not list Complex PTSD as a diagnosis, the World Health Organization's *International Classification of Diseases* (ICD-10) recognized this experience as different from PTSD, calling it Enduring Personality Change After Catastrophic Experience (EPCACE; Reed et al., 2022). In the 11th version (ICD-11), this changed to Complex Posttraumatic Stress Disorder (WHO, 2022). Despite this recognition, many providers were slow to recognize or use this diagnosis with clients or patients. Earlier, the *DSM-IV* committee was considering a new diagnosis called complex PTSD (Herman, 1992), which was alternatively named DESNOS, a Disorder of Extreme Stress Not Otherwise Specified (Van der Kolk et al., 2005). Some individuals experienced PTSD symptoms, emotion regulation difficulties, a negative self-concept, and interpersonal disturbance. The World Health Organization considered and included Complex PTSD (C-PTSD), recognizing the core symptoms of PTSD and the core features of the three domains of emotion regulation difficulties, negative self-concept, and interpersonal distress (Reed et al., 2022). This inclusion resulted from research studies showing that some with chronic PTSD symptoms, multiple traumas, and enduring personality changes needed a diagnosis beyond PTSD (Reed et al., 2022).

This diagnosis is a debatable topic as some professionals do not consider it a distinctive diagnosis from PTSD and instead view it as a severe type of PTSD, a prolonged grief reaction, conversion disorder, or a histrionic disorder. Other professionals view it as posttraumatic embitterment or an adjustment disorder (Lindauer et al., 2023). While the *DSM-5-TR* committee considered inclusion, they did not include it because of little empirical evidence (VA, 2024b). The primary reasons for the lack of inclusion were the lack of a consistent definition, the lack of standardized and validated measures for the condition, and the difficulty in differentiating the diagnosis from borderline personality disorder (Resick et al., 2012). However, the World Health Organization took a different approach to the *ICD-11*. It included it as a diagnosis after conducting two global surveys of over 3,000 psychiatrists and psychologists from 35 countries

Searching for a Diagnosis

who suggested including the diagnosis. The WHO determined that the concerns of the diagnosis were addressable since numerous studies supported the diagnosis (Brewin et al., 2017).

In the *ICD-11*, PTSD comprises exposure to an event or repeated events that are threatening or horrifying, including those that are extended or repetitive and from which escape is difficult or impossible (WHO, 2022). The *ICD-11* states that the following three core elements of PTSD must be present for at least several weeks:

- Experiencing the traumatic event(s) again, which may include vivid intrusive memories or pictures, flashbacks, or recurring dreams or nightmares associated with the trauma. The process of re-experiencing requires the presence of profound or overpowering emotions and acute bodily sensations. Mere contemplation or recollection of the event, along with recalling one's encounter at that moment, is inadequate to fulfill the need of reexperiencing.
- Conscious effort to avoid thoughts, memories, actions, or any other reminders of the occurrence, both internally and externally, including avoiding discussions, persons, locations, or anything else associated with the event.
- Sustained beliefs of increased present danger, such as excessive vigilance or an apparent alteration in one's reaction to sudden stimuli, may be intensified or reduced.

(WHO, 2022)

Furthermore, the *ICD-11* states that C-PTSD includes three symptom categories of self-organization (DSO) disturbances: affective dysregulation, negative self-concept, and interpersonal relationship difficulties (WHO, 2022).

- The individual experiences severe and persistent difficulties regulating their emotions, characterized by an exaggerated emotional response to mild stimuli, frequent emotional outbursts, prospective or actual self-harming behavior, detachment from reality, emotional numbness, or an inability to feel pleasure or good feelings.
- Chronic and enduring convictions of diminished self-worth, personal defeat, or insignificance, accompanied by feelings of shame, guilt, or inadequacy.
- Chronic difficulties in maintaining relationships or experiencing emotional intimacy. The individual may purposefully evade or have minimal interest

in emotional connection with others or, if it does occur, struggle to sustain enduring connections.

(VA, 2024b; WHO, 2022)

While the focus of C-PTSD is related to childhood trauma, other traumatic events include long-term domestic violence, concentration camps, prisoner-of-war camps, prostitution rings, and long-term child physical abuse. Research suggests that the intensity and duration of trauma account for the additional symptoms (VA, 2024b). In the conceptualization of treatment or aid for people with C-PTSD symptoms, one must build trust due to the extensive harm that occurred over time. C-PTSD frequently coexists with various mental health issues like alcohol use disorders, dissociative disorders, depressive disorders, and anxiety disorders. While the prevalence of PTSD shows a higher rate for women than men and middle-aged adults over older adults, the C-PTSD rates are equivalent for men and women and are not lower among older adults (Maercker et al., 2022).

While some acknowledge C-PTSD as a possible condition, other researchers have proposed Developmental Trauma Disorder as a diagnosis. This syndrome, resembling PTSD, is associated with childhood trauma and is connected to physical assault, abuse, domestic violence, emotional abuse, separation from caregivers, disability, and multiple traumatic events. Developmental trauma disorder is like complex posttraumatic stress disorder (C-PTSD), but it also acknowledges the impact of childhood and adolescence on the development of the disorder. The diagnosis was proposed for inclusion in the *DSM-5* but was rejected due to a lack of empirical evidence (Spinazzola et al., 2021).

As stated previously, traumatized individuals may have symptoms that meet the criteria for Acute Stress Disorder or PTSD. Those with multiple or prolonged childhood trauma may have C-PTSD and yet be diagnosed with PTSD. Others who experience trauma may have posttraumatic symptoms that resolve quickly or do not cause moderate to severe impairment in functioning. Others may not meet the full criteria for diagnosis but experience problems in personal, educational, or occupational performance. Sometimes, people are diagnosed with other mental health conditions due to the lack of a comprehensive assessment. Alternatively, an individual may have PTSD and another mental health condition. The mental health condition may be present prior to trauma exposure, develop because of trauma exposure, or co-occur with PTSD. It is essential to understand the most common conditions that may occur or may be mistakenly assigned.

Searching for a Diagnosis

Co-occurring Disorders or Confounded with Trauma Diagnoses

Determining whether someone has a trauma diagnosis or another mental health condition can be challenging. The stressor- or trauma-related diagnoses may be confused with depressive disorders, anxiety disorders, or personality disorders, such as borderline personality disorder. In such cases, further clarification and a general understanding of these other mental health conditions may be needed. One of the key elements will be the inquiry into the present, recent, or history of trauma. It is common for patients or clients to receive a diagnosis of another mental disorder, such as depression or anxiety, instead of acute stress disorder, PTSD, or C-PTSD (Gagnon-Sanschagrin et al., 2022). PTSD often goes undiagnosed in both military and civilian adults because of misdiagnosis, lack of awareness of trauma-related conditions, patients not disclosing their experiences, or clinicians failing to inquire about trauma (Schein et al., 2021). Knowing the criteria of other disorders and how the confusion occurs is helpful even if your job is not as a diagnostician.

Depressive Disorders

The *DSM-5-TR* categorizes depressive disorders into nine distinct types. These are Disruptive Mood Dysregulation Disorder, Major Depressive Disorder, Persistent Depressive Disorder, Premenstrual Dysphoric Disorder, Substance/Medication-Induced Depressive Disorder, Depressive Disorder Due to Another Medical Condition, Other Specified Depressive Disorder, Unspecified Depressive Disorder, and Unspecified Mood Disorder (APA, 2022). The dilemma arises when a person experiences co-occurring symptoms in these conditions and trauma-related disorders. The first step for all helping professionals is recognizing that many disorders have overlapping symptoms. When a person experiences a mental health disorder, it can also impact their ability to report symptoms, the onset, duration, and changes.

There is no room to describe the nine distinct types of depressive disorders. Instead, this chapter focuses on the differential diagnosis of major depressive disorder and PTSD. All depressive disorders include sadness, emptiness, irritable mood, and related factors that affect a person's ability to function. The differences between these disorders are duration, timing, or etiology, which explain the pre-existing factors that cause or lead to a depressed condition (APA, 2022). Symptoms of major depressive disorder include symptoms that persist for a minimum of two weeks and include noticeable alterations in mood, thinking, and daily functioning. The symptoms must encompass at least one indication of a despondent mood, diminished capacity for experiencing interest, or typical pleasure gained from daily life.

Furthermore, an individual may also undergo substantial fluctuations in body weight, either losing or gaining, as well as a decrease or increase in appetite. They may also experience disruptions in their sleep patterns, either struggling to fall asleep or experiencing excessive restlessness. Additionally, they may exhibit psychomotor agitation or retardation, where their physical movements are either excessively fast or slowed down. They may also experience persistent fatigue or a loss of energy, along with feelings of worthlessness or excessive and inappropriate guilt. Their ability to concentrate and make decisions may be significantly impaired. Lastly, they may have recurrent thoughts of death. The symptoms result in substantial distress or impairment in critical aspects of life, such as work, relationships, or other vital areas. Additionally, the physiological effects of a substance or any other medical condition do not cause the symptoms (APA, 2022). Several of these symptoms share similarities with PTSD, including anhedonia, sleep disruption, heightened anger, attention difficulties, and feelings of guilt (VA, 2024c).

In epidemiological studies, approximately 50% of people with PTSD also have a diagnosis of major depressive disorder. However, distinct biological factors differentiate the two conditions. In neuroimaging, major depressive disorder and PTSD show differences with lower hippocampal volume and higher activity in the dorsal anterior cingulate cortex in PTSD. This suggests that threats more highly activate people with PTSD. There is also a distinction between the hypothalamic–pituitary–adrenal (HPA) axis functioning with lower peripheral cortisol levels in PTSD but higher in major depressive disorder. An individual can indeed experience multiple mental health disorders. Researchers hypothesize that the two diagnoses interact (Flory & Yehuda, 2015). In a longitudinal study, patients diagnosed with comorbid PTSD and major depressive disorder had persistent symptoms for up to six years after initial screening than those diagnosed with PTSD or major depressive disorder alone (Armenta et al., 2019).

Bipolar and Related Disorders

Bipolar and Related Disorders can co-occur with trauma-related disorders. These include Bipolar I and Bipolar II Disorder, Cyclothymic Disorder, Substance/Medication-Induced Bipolar Disorder, Bipolar Disorder Due to Another Medical Condition,

Other Specified Bipolar and Related Disorders, Unspecified Bipolar Disorder, and Unspecified Mood Disorder (APA, 2022). When considering whether a person may have PTSD or bipolar disorder, the helper should know that these diagnoses can both be present (Cogan et al., 2020). Between 6 and 55% of adults with PTSD also met the criteria for bipolar disorder, and between 4 and 40% diagnosed with bipolar disorder met the criteria for PTSD (Cerimele et al., 2017). It may be that people with bipolar disorder have higher frequency rates of childhood abuse or neglect and a higher risk of developing PTSD (Cogan et al., 2020). The symptoms of bipolar disorder encompass an elevated, expansive, or irritable mood, heightened goal-directed activity, inflated self-esteem or grandiosity, increased talkativeness or pressured speech, flight of ideas, psychomotor agitation, feeling rested despite minimal sleep, recurrent thoughts of death, psychomotor retardation or agitation, significant changes in weight or appetite, and fatigue or loss of energy. The shared symptoms of bipolar illness and PTSD encompass disrupted sleep patterns, impaired capacity to focus, heightened propensity for risk-taking, loss of pleasure in activities, feelings of guilt, heightened anger, and enduring negative emotional states (APA, 2022). Using a formal clinical interview and a trauma-screening instrument is helpful in determining which is present or both.

Anxiety Disorders

In previous editions of the *DSM*, PTSD was listed as an anxiety-related disorder. However, in the *DSM-5-TR*, PTSD is now listed as a trauma- and stressor-related disorder (APA, 2022). This reclassification was because of considerable research that provided evidence of emotions such as guilt, shame, and anger that were not part of the fear or anxiety classification (Pai et al., 2017). However, PTSD and anxiety-related disorders commonly share symptoms such as fear, disrupted sleep, and difficulty concentrating. The *DSM-5-TR* includes a comprehensive list of anxiety disorders, which consists of separation anxiety disorder, selective mutism, specific phobia, social anxiety disorder, panic disorder, agoraphobia, generalized anxiety disorder, substance/medication-induced anxiety disorder, anxiety disorder due to another medical condition, and other specified anxiety disorder (APA, 2022). In the absence of a trauma screening or a comprehensive clinical interview, a person with PTSD may appear to have a generalized anxiety disorder or a specific phobia (Levin-Aspenson et al., 2021). Lab examination reveals disparities in inflammatory markers between PTSD and anxiety-related disorders (Williamson et al., 2021).

Some experts argue that a differential diagnosis is possible through a trauma screening and clinical interview. During this process, the helper can seek the specific core symptoms of PTSD, such as reexperiencing the traumatic event and avoidance symptoms (Rasmussen et al., 2019). However, other researchers argue that other disorders also share these symptoms (Lockwood & Forbes, 2014). Reexperiencing that includes a thought disorder could be a psychotic symptom, whereas avoidance is a common feature of specific phobia (Levin-Aspenson et al., 2021). Without a doubt, grasping the overlap is essential.

Personality Disorders

Distinguishing a trauma-related diagnosis, in particular C-PTSD, from a personality disorder such as borderline personality disorder is essential. A personality disorder refers to a persistent pattern of internal feelings and behaviors that significantly diverge from the accepted cultural standards and expectations. These traits are enduring and inflexible, maintaining stability throughout an individual's lifetime, and causing distress or impairment in one or multiple aspects of life (APA, 2022). Three clusters, A, B, and C, classify ten personality disorders. These clusters do not encompass a personality disorder resulting from another medical condition or a specified or unspecified personality disorder where the symptoms are present but lack distinguishable characteristics or sufficient information for diagnosis. The ten types included in the *DSM-5-TR* include paranoid, schizoid, schizotypal, antisocial, borderline, histrionic, narcissistic, avoidant, dependent, and obsessive-compulsive personality disorder, not to be confused with obsessive-compulsive disorder (APA, 2022). Approximately 12% of individuals in Western countries have a personality disorder. The highest prevalence was obsessive-compulsive personality disorder, and the lowest was dependent personality disorder (Volkert et al., 2018). The prevalence of borderline personality disorder in the U.S. is between 0.7% and 2.7% of adults. However, prevalence rates are higher among patients in outpatient clinical settings and psychiatric hospitals (Ellison et al., 2018).

A common concern about C-PTSD is the symptom overlap between this trauma-related disorder and borderline personality disorder. This is because affective instability, impulse control, and difficulty in relationships are evident in both. Some argue that a well-defined distinction is lacking (Resick et al., 2012). Borderline personality disorder (BPD) encompasses symptoms related to a strong fear of being abandoned,

Searching for a Diagnosis

unstable and intense relationships, a disturbed sense of identity, a feeling of emptiness, impulsive behavior, repeated suicidal or self-harming actions like cutting, emotional instability including intense and inappropriate anger, and temporary experiences of paranoia or dissociation during times of stress (APA, 2022). While some state that borderline personality disorder is related to childhood trauma, this is not true for all diagnosed with the condition. There is insufficient evidence yet to state a neurobiological difference, except for a hyperactive amygdala (Peled-Avron et al., 2020). Diagnosing a person with borderline personality disorder can sometimes result in misdiagnosis or the coexistence of C-PTSD. If trauma history exists, then diagnosing C-PTSD may be less stigmatizing and more accurate than diagnosing BPD (Ford & Courtois, 2021). This conceptualization may be more helpful in determining the best course of treatment.

Tending Your Technique

Elizabeth, a 55-year-old female teacher, comes for help due to her problem sustaining long-term relationships with family and friends. She wants to know if she has borderline personality disorder or other personality disorders. At times, Elizabeth has been suicidal and has attempted to harm herself. She does not like pain, so she did not hurt herself for long. However, Elizabeth was promiscuous as a young adult, often offering her body to receive attention for a short while. As she tells one story after another, you notice themes of affective dysregulation and a poor self-image. Elizabeth blames herself for most of the damage in her relationships. Elizabeth shares some distressful experiences, including being physically and sexually abused by her father, raped by a priest, being laid off, and a terrible work event that led to her suspension. When you ask about her background, Elizabeth shares the story of her biological father's alcoholism, physical abuse of her mother, and emotional abuse of the children. While Elizabeth was relatively young when her parents divorced, she has a clear memory of specific times with her father that were disturbing. This is your case. Answer these questions.

- How would you decide whether Elizabeth has a borderline personality disorder or a trauma-related diagnosis?
- What symptoms are present in this case that helped you decide?
- What further information do you need?

Awareness of how PTSD may be underdiagnosed and maybe a comorbid condition, guides you in providing trauma-informed care. While you may not diagnose these conditions or feel comfortable doing so, you can understand how difficult it may be for other professionals to determine which and how many diagnoses are present, particularly when symptoms overlap or symptoms are absent.

A Flourishing Focus

While a person who experiences a trauma may develop mild, moderate, or severe symptoms, many individuals, possibly up to 88%, do not develop or have long-lasting deleterious effects (Zheng et al., 2020). This leads us to question how that can be. Are people born with protective genetic factors? That may be possible. Some studies indicate that lower amygdala activation is linked to higher resilience and better responses to stress stimuli (Barbour et al., 2020). Other studies indicate higher resilience with lower spontaneous activity and global functional connectivity in the default mode network (Altinok et al., 2021).

Could it be that people do not develop PTSD or other diagnoses because of their personality types? There is a correlation between highly resilient people and certain personality traits. People who are more extroverted or engaged with the outer world tend to have more positive emotions; those who are conscientious, in other words, self-disciplined, organized, and responsible, tend to score higher in resilience. On the other hand, individuals who have high levels of neuroticism, or the tendency to interpret situations as threatening, or have frequent negative emotions, tend to score lower in resilience (Altinok et al., 2021).

Some hypothesize that cultural differences explain the variances in whether or not one develops PTSD. If resilience refers to psychological adjustment after trauma, one's self-construal may matter. In Western cultures, people tend to be independent, focusing on being separate and unique. Having an independent self-construal means one might be more likely to ruminate on autobiographic memories of traumatic experiences, thus leading to negative attributions and interpretations of events. In Eastern cultures, by contrast, an interdependent self-construal is encouraged with connectedness and reliance upon community. Interdependence occurs with the support of the community. A third view is from Chinese culture, which is a dialecticism-oriented one.

Viewing life as both negative and positive, passive and active, feminine and masculine, enables one to tolerate inconsistencies that arise in situations, thoughts, and emotions (Ali et al., 2023; Raghavan & Sandanapitchai, 2024; Zheng et al., 2020).

According to the salutogenic model, based on the sense of coherence, learned experiences and identification of general and specific resistance resources can act as protectors or, at the least, diminish trauma effects. These general resistance resources may be coping skills learned during childhood and adolescence, personality characteristics, or community influences (Schäfer et al., 2019). Whether higher resilience results from neurobiological differences, personality characteristics, cultural differences, or general resistance resources, it demonstrates further need for exploring why people do not develop more symptoms that impair functioning. With such, we might be able to identify ways to protect individuals from the adverse effects of trauma.

While diagnoses are essential for determining a treatment pathway, sometimes they can cause stigmatization or discourage those with trauma experiences. In our work, we remind one another and our students that when we encounter someone who has been through a traumatic event, they are a person first, not a disorder. This is part of trauma sensitivity. Mistaking behaviors and symptoms, inferring a person is a disease or dysfunctional person, dishonors their essential humanness. Before we adopted this view, we heard a leader say, "Everyone is creative, resourceful, and whole." We tried to argue that might not be true. We were mistaken as time passed, and as we have changed our concept, focusing on the person first gives them courage and strength and aids us in providing trauma-sensitive care. The best part is "Finding the gems among the rocks." In other words, look for what is good, kind, and healthy. Explore the person's strengths and help them grow in their resilience.

Gather Self-Awareness

- Please describe what you learned about diagnosis in this chapter and how it affects you.
- As you reflect on your own experiences with trauma or those close to you who have endured difficulties, what do you believe affected how they were affected?

Chapter Summary

This chapter aimed to ensure that all professionals working with traumatized individuals have an initial introduction and understanding of trauma diagnoses and case conceptualization. Whether you are a mental health provider, teacher, nurse, or emergency personnel, understanding trauma effects and developing sensitivity will provide a more focused approach and offer safety to those experiencing trauma. An understanding of the subtle differences in trauma-related stress disorders, such as acute stress disorder, posttraumatic stress disorder, and complex-post-traumatic stress disorder, is vital to determine the best course of treatment. The chapter discusses how these trauma-related disorders may be misdiagnosed as other mental health disorders, such as depression, anxiety disorders, or personality disorders, when they may be comorbid conditions. Finally, the chapter offers a reminder to view people holistically, using a trauma-sensitive approach.

Chapter Review

Please respond to the following questions.

1. What are some potential challenges in diagnosing trauma-related stress disorders?
2. How can trauma-related disorders be comorbid with other mental health conditions?
3. What other mental health conditions may be comorbid or mistaken as the primary diagnosis?
4. How can you incorporate a salutogenic approach in diagnosing people?

Key Term Assessment

Review the following terms and try to explain each concept.

- Acute Stress Disorder
- Posttraumatic Stress Disorder
- Complex-Post Traumatic Stress Disorder

Resources

The following resources may be helpful. At the time of this writing, they were accessible through the links provided.

- CPTSD Foundation helps with healing and trauma recovery through therapy networks, coaching, legal services, and research.
- The National Institute for the Clinical Application of Behavioral Medicine (NICABM) offers training and education on trauma, treatments for trauma, and research.
- U.S. Department of Veterans Affairs. PTSD: National Center for PTSD. This site is the world's leading research and educational center on PTSD. It offers practical advice, access to resources, and helpful information about traumatic stress disorders.

References

Ali, D. A., Figley, C. R., Tedeschi, R. G., Galarneau, D., & Amara, S. (2023). Shared trauma, resilience, and growth: A roadmap toward transcultural conceptualization. *Psychological Trauma: Theory, Research, Practice, and Policy, 15*(1), 45–55. https://doi.org/10.1037/tra0001044

Altinok, D. C. A., Rajkumar, R., Nießen, D., Sbaihat, H., Kersey, M., Shah, N. J., Vesselinović, T., & Neuner, I. (2021). Common neurobiological correlates of resilience and personality traits within the triple resting-state brain networks assessed by 7-Tesla ultra-high field MRI. *Scientific Reports, 11*, 11564. https://doi.org/10.1038/s41598-021-91056-y

American Psychiatric Association. (1980). *The diagnostic and statistical manual for mental disorders* (*DSM-III*). American Psychiatric Association.

American Psychiatric Association. (1994). *The diagnostic and statistical manual for mental disorders* (*DSM-IV-TR*). American Psychiatric Association.

American Psychiatric Association. (2022). *The diagnostic and statistical manual for mental disorders fifth edition text revision* (*DSM-5-TR*). American Psychiatric Association.

Armenta, R. F., Walter, K. H., Geronimo-Hara, T. R., Porter, B., Stander, V. A., & LeardMann, C. A. (2019). Longitudinal trajectories of comorbid PTSD and depression symptoms among U.S. service members and veterans. *BMC Psychiatry, 19*, 396. https://doi.org/10.1186/s12888-019-2375-1

Barbour, T., Holmes, A. J., Farabaugh, A. H., DeCross, S. N., Coombs, G., Boeke, E. A., Wolthusen, R. P. F., Nyer, M., Pedrelli, P., Fava, M., & Holt, D. J. (2020). Elevated amygdala activity in young adults with familial risk for depression: A potential marker of low resilience. *Biological Psychiatry: Cognitive Neuroscience and Neuroimaging, 5*(2), 194–202. https://doi.org/10.1016/j.bpsc.2019.10.010

Ben-Ezra, M. (2004). Trauma in antiquity: 4000 year old posttraumatic reactions? *Stress & Health, 20*(3), 121–125. https://doi.org/10.1002/smi.1003

Birmes, P., Hatton, L., Brunet, A., & Schmitt, L. (2003). Early historical literature for posttraumatic symptomatology. *Stress & Health, 19*(1), 17–26. https://doi.org/10.1002/smi.952

Brewin, C. R., Coitre, M., Hyland, P., Shevlin, M., Maercker, A., Bryant, R. A., Humayun, A., Jones, L. M., Kagee, A., Rousseau, C., Somasundaram, D., Suzuki, Y., Wessely, S., van Ommeren, M., & Reed, G. (2017). A review of current evidence regarding the ICD-11 proposals for diagnosing PTSD and complex PTSD. *Clinical Psychology Review, 58*, 1–15. https://doi.org/10.1016/j.cpr.2017.09.001

Bryant, R. A. (2023). Controversies in posttraumatic stress disorder. In C. L. Cobb, S. J. Lynn, & W. O'Donohue (Eds.), *Toward a science of clinical psychology*. Springer.

Bryant, R. A., Friedman, M. J., Spiegal, D., Ursano, R., & Strain, J. (2011). A review of acute stress disorder in *DSM-5*. *Depression and Anxiety, 28*(9), 802–817. https://doi.org/10.1002/da.20737

Campodonico, C., Berry, K., Haddock, G., & Varese, F. (2021). Protective factors associated with posttraumatic outcomes in individuals with experiences of psychosis. *Frontiers in Psychiatry, 12*, 735870. https://doi.org/10.3389/fpsyt.2021.735870

Cardeña, E., & Carlson, E. (2011). Acute stress disorder revisited. *Annual Review of Clinical Psychology, 7*, 245–267. https://doi.org/10.1146/annurev-clinpsy-032210-104502

Carlson, E. B., Palmieri, P. A., Field, N. P., Dalenberg, C. J., Macia, K. S., & Spain, D. A. (2016). Contributions of risk and protective factors to prediction of psychological symptoms after traumatic experiences. *Comprehensive Psychiatry, 69*, 106–115. https://doi.org/10.1016/j.comppsych.2016.04.022

Cerimele, J. M., Bauer, A. M., Fortney, J. C., & Bauer, M. S. (2017). Patients with co-occurring bipolar disorder and posttraumatic stress disorder: A rapid review of the literature. *The Journal of Clinical Psychiatry, 78*(5), e506–e514. https://doi.org/10.40088/jcp.16r10897

Cogan, C. M., Paquet, C. B., Lee, J. Y., Miller, K. E., Crowley, M. D., & Davis, J. L. (2020). Differentiating the symptoms of posttraumatic stress disorder and bipolar disorders in adults: Utilizing a trauma-informed assessment approach. *Clinical Psychology & Psychotherapy, 28*(1). https://doi.org/10.1002/cpp2504

References

Ellison, W. D., Rosenstein, L. K., Morga, T. A., & Zimmerman, M. (2018). Community and clinical epidemiology of borderline personality disorder. *Psychiatric Clinics of North America, 41*(4), 561–573. https://doi.org/10.1016/j.psc.2018.07.008

Fanai, M., & Khan, M. A. B. (2024). *Acute stress disorder.* StatPearls. https://www.ncbi.nlm.nih.gov/books/NBK560815/

Flory, J. D., & Yehuda, R. (2015). Comorbidity between posttraumatic stress disorder and major depressive disorder: Alternative explanations and treatment considerations. *Dialogues in Clinical Neuroscience, 17*(2), 141–150. https://doi.org/10.31887/DCNS.2015.17.2/jflory

Ford, J. D., & Courtois, C. A. (2021). Complex PTSD and borderline personality disorder. *Borderline Personality Disorder and Emotion Dysregulation, 8*(16). https://doi.org/10.1186/s40479-021-00155-9

Friedman, M. J. (2023). *PTSD history and overview.* PTSD: National Center for PTSD.

Friedman, M. J., Schnurr, P. P., & Keane, T. M. (2021). PTSD from DSM-III to DSM-5: Progress and challenges. In M. J. Friedman, P. P. Schnurr, & T. M. Keane (Eds.), *Handbook of PTSD: Science and practice* (pp. 3–18). Guilford Publications.

Gagnon-Sanschagrin, P., Schein, J., Urganus, A., Serra, E., Liang, Y., Musingarimi, P., Cloutier, M., Guérin, A., & Davis, L. L. (2022). Identifying individuals with undiagnosed posttraumatic stress disorder in a large United States civilian population—a machine learning approach. *BMC Psychiatry, 22*, 630. https://doi.org/10.1186/s12888-022-04267-6

Gentry, J. E., Baranowsky, A. B., & Rhoton, R. (2017). Trauma competency: An active ingredient approach to treating posttraumatic stress disorder. *Journal of Counseling & Development, 95*(3), 245–366. https://aztrauma.org/wp-content/uploads/2018/01/Trauma-Competency-JCD.pdf

Geoffrion, S., Goncalves, J., Robichaud, I., Sader, J., Giguère, C.-É., Fortin, M., Lamothe, J., Bernard, P., & Guay, S. (2022). Systematic review and meta-analysis on acute stress disorder: Rates following different types of traumatic events. *Trauma, Violence, & Abuse, 23*(1), 213–223. https://doi.org/10.1177/1524838020933844

Henninger, J. (2021). Protective and risk factors associated with posttraumatic growth and psychopathological symptoms following trauma. (Publication No. 541) [Doctoral dissertation, Philadelphia College of Osteopathic Medicine]. PCOM Psychology Dissertations.

Herman, J. L. (1992). *Trauma and recovery: The aftermath of violence from domestic violence to political terrorism.* Guilford.

Kramer, L. (2016). Familial betrayal and trauma in select plays of Shakespeare, Racine, and the Corneilles. [Doctoral dissertation]. University of South Carolina.

Kucmin, T., Kucmin, A., Nogalski, A., Sojczuk, S., & Jojczuk, M. (2016). History of trauma and posttraumatic disorders in literature. *Psychiatria Polska, 50*(1), 269–281. https://doi.org/10.12740/PP/43039

Levin-Aspenson, H. F., & Greene, A. L. (2024). Rethinking trauma-related psychopathology in the Hierarchical Taxonomy of Psychopathology (HiTOP). *Journal of Traumatic Stress*, 1–11. https://doi.org/10.1002/jts.23014

Levin-Aspenson, H. F., Watson, D., Ellickson-Larew, S., Stanton, K., & Stasik-O'Brien, S. M. (2021). Beyond distress and fear: Differential psychopathology correlates of PTSD symptom clusters. *Journal of Affective Disorders*, *284*, 9–17. https://doi.org/10.1016/j.jad.2021.01.090

Lindauer, M., Linden, M., & Muschalla, B. (2023). Conceptualization of stress-related disorders and PTSD by cognitive behavior therapists. *Verhaltenstherapie*. https://doi.org/10.1159/000527652

Lockwood, E., & Forbes, D. (2014). Posttraumatic stress disorder and comorbidity: Untangling the Gordian knot. *Psychological Injury and Law*, *7*, 108–121. https://doi.org/10.1007/s12207-014-9189-8

Maercker, A., Cloitre, M., Bachem, R., Schlumpf, Y. R., Khoury, B., Hitchcock, C., & Bohus, M. (2022). Complex posttraumatic stress disorder. *The Lancet*, *400*(10345), 60–72. https://doi.org/10.1016/S0140-6736(22)00821-2

Mambrol, N. (2018, July 15). *Trauma studies*. Literary Theory and Criticism.

Marshall, R. D., Olfson, M., Hellman, F., Blanco, C., Guardino, M., & Struening, E. L. (2001). Comorbidity, impairment, and suicidality in subthreshold PTSD. *American Journal of Psychiatry*, *158*(9), 1467–1473. https://doi.org/10.1176/appi.ajp.158.9.1467

Micale, M. S. (1995). Charcot and *les névroses traumatiques*: Scientific and historical reflections. *Journal of the History of the Neurosciences*, *4*(2), 101–119. https://doi.org/10.1080/09647049509525630

Pai, A., Suris, A. M., & North, C. S. (2017). Posttraumatic stress disorder in the DSM-5: Controversy, change, and conceptual considerations. *Behavioral Sciences (Basel, Switzerland)*, *7*(1), 7. https://doi.org/10.3390/bs7010007

Peled-Avron, L., Abu-Akel, A., & Shamay-Tsoory, S. (2020). Exogenous effects of oxytocin in five psychiatric disorders: A systematic review, meta-analyses and a personalized approach through the lens of the social salience hypothesis. *Neuroscience and Biobehavioral Reviews*, *114*, 70–95. https://doi.org/10.1016/j.neubiorev.2020.04.023

Pinel, P. (1797). *Nosographie philosophique*. De l'impr. de Crapelet.

Raghavan, S., & Sandanapitchai, P. (2024). The relationship between cultural variables and resilience to psychological trauma: A systematic review of the literature. *Traumatology*, *30*(1), 37–51. https://doi.org/10.1037/trm0000239

Rasmussen, A., Verkuilen, J., Jayawickreme, N., Wu, Z., & McCluskey, S. T. (2019). When did posttraumatic stress disorder get so many factors? Confirmatory factor models since *DSM-5*. *Clinical Psychological Science*, *7*(2). https://doi.org/10.1177/2167702618809370

Reed, G. M., First, M. B., Billieux, J., Cloitre, M., Briken, P., Achab, S., Brewin, C. R., King, D. L., Kraus, S. W., & Bryant, R. A. (2022). Emerging experience with selected new categories in the *ICD-11*: Complex PTSD, prolonged grief disorder, gaming disorder, and compulsive sexual behaviour disorder. *World Psychiatry, 21*(2), 189–213. https://doi.org/10.1002/wps.20960

Resick, P. A., Bovin, M. J., Calloway, A. L., Dick, A. M., King, M. W., Mitchell, K. S., Suvak, M. K., Wells, S. Y., Stirman, S. W., & Wolf, E. J. (2012). A critical evaluation of the complex PTSD literature: Implications for DSM-5. *Journal of Traumatic Stress, 25*(3), 241–251. https://doi.org/10.1002/jts.21699

Schäfer, S. K., Becker, N., King, L., Horsch, A., & Michael, T. (2019). The relationship between sense of coherence and posttraumatic stress: A meta-analysis. *European Journal of Psychotraumatology, 10*(1). https://doi.org/10.1080/20008198.2018.1562839

Scheeringa, M. (2023). *PTSD for children 6 years and younger*. PTSD: National Center for PTSD. https://www.ptsd.va.gov/professional/treat/specific/ptsd_child_under6.asp

Schein, J., Houle, C., Urganus, A., Cloutier, M., Patterson-Lomba, O., Wang, Y., King, S., Levinson, W., Guérin, A., Lefebvre, P., & Davis, L. L. (2021). Prevalence of posttraumatic stress disorder in the United States: A systematic literature review. *Current Medical Research and Opinion, 37*(12), 2151–2161. https://doi.org/10.1080/03007995.2021.1978417

Schultebraucks, K., Sijbrandij, M., Galatzer-Levy, I., Mouthaan, J., Olff, M., & van Zuiden, M. (2021). Forecasting individual risk for long-term posttraumatic stress disorder in emergency medical settings using biomedical data: A machine learning multicenter cohort study. *Neurobiology of Stress, 14*, 100297. https://doi.org/10.1016/j.ynstr.2021.100297

Spiers, T., & Harrington, G. (2001). A brief history of trauma (ch. 8). In Spiers, T. (Ed.), *Trauma*. Routledge.

Spinazzola, J., Van der Kolk, B., & Ford, J. D. (2021). Developmental trauma disorder: A legacy of attachment trauma in victimized children. *Journal of Traumatic Stress, 34*(4), 711–720. https://doi.org/10.1002/jts.22697

Substance Abuse and Mental Health Services Administration (SAMHSA). (2014). *Treatment improvement protocol* (TIP series, No. 57). Center for Substance Abuse Treatment.

U.S. Department of Veterans Affairs (VA). (2024a). *Acute stress disorder*. PTSD: National Center for PTSD.

U.S. Department of Veterans Affairs (VA). (2024b). *Complex PTSD*. PTSD: National Center for PTSD.

U.S. Department of Veterans Affairs (VA). (2024c). *Depression, trauma, and PTSD*. PTSD: National Center for PTSD.

Van der Kolk, B. A., Roth, S., Pelcovitz, D., Sunday, S., & Spinazzola, J. (2005). Disorders of extreme stress: The empirical foundation of a complex adaptation to trauma. *Journal of Traumatic Stress, 18*(5), 389–399. https://doi.org/10.1002/jts.20047

Volkert, J., Gablonski, T. C., & Rabung, S. (2018). Prevalence of personality disorders in the general adult population in Western countries: Systematic review and meta-analysis. *The British Journal of Psychiatry, 213*(6), 709–713. https://doi.org/10.1192/bjp.2018.202

Williamson, J. B., Jaffee, M. S., & Jorge, R. E. (2021). Posttraumatic stress disorder and anxiety-related conditions. *Behavioral Neurology and Psychiatry, 27*(6), 1738–1763. https://doi.org/10.1212/CON.0000000000001054

World Health Organization (WHO). (1999). *The international classification of diseases* (10th ed.). https://www.cdc.gov/nchs/icd/icd-10-cm.htm

World Health Organization (WHO). (2022). *The international classification of diseases* (11th ed.). https://www.cdc.gov/nchs/icd/icd-10-cm.htm

Zheng, P., Gray, M. J., Duan, W.-J., Ho, S. M. Y., Xia, M., & Clapp, J. D. (2020). An exploration of the relationship between culture and resilience capacity in trauma survivors. *Journal of Cross-Cultural Psychology, 51*(6), 407–527. https://doi.org/10.1177/0022022120925907

Chapter Six
Evidence-Based Treatments

Overview

Chapter 6: Evidence-Based Treatments discusses the terms trauma-sensitive approaches, trauma-informed approaches, trauma-informed care, trauma-specific services, and trauma-informed practice. It provides established guidelines from the Veterans Administration, the American Psychological Association, the National Institute for Health and Care Excellence, and the International Society for Traumatic Stress Studies on the treatment of trauma and PTSD. The most recommended evidence-based psychotherapy treatments for adults are explained. Additionally, the chapter discusses treatments focused on children and adolescents, including parent education programs. The chapter concludes with a discussion of resilience and posttraumatic growth.

Treating Trauma

Professional service to others means a helper must understand how to provide trauma-informed care and what people encounter in their post-trauma life. People who experience painful events may feel powerless and challenged in their worldview. They may doubt who they are and their ability to function in life or move to a rewarding existence. These people may have difficulty making sense of the world or trusting others (Kleber, 2019). This disequilibrium is due to the loss of control and vulnerability caused by traumatic events. Janoff-Bulman (1992) states that a person's view of themselves and the world around them no longer fits previous conceptions. Whatever assumptions one had are now profoundly altered.

DOI: 10.4324/9781003463009-6

Knowing what to do, how to help, and when to provide trauma services is more complex than one realizes and, therefore, entails learning fundamental information before helping. Many individuals who encounter a traumatic event will not develop a mental health disorder like PTSD. However, they may exhibit posttraumatic stress symptoms (van der Velden et al., 2006). Indications may include trouble sleeping, mood swings, changes in appetite, intrusive thoughts, or avoiding reminders of the incident. They may sense that no one else can understand their devastating event, resulting in estrangement from others. However, these symptoms may not rise above a threshold level that meets the criteria for Acute Stress Disorder or PTSD (APA, 2022).

Family, friends, colleagues, community, or professionals can provide valuable support to those with trauma. In studies of disasters, social support appears to buffer the development of severe symptoms. Multiple studies have shown the value of social encouragement in reducing adverse mental health outcomes, enhancing recovery, and reducing posttraumatic stress symptoms (APA, 2022; Danielson et al., 2017; Fredette et al., 2016). However, when such help is unavailable, there is a significant risk of emerging mental health disorders (Dückers, 2017; Fredette et al., 2016). A provider's connection with a distressed person can positively impact the traumatized individual. This contextual model is a dominant framework describing the common factors among all trauma approaches. It shows how the bond between a helper and a client increases hope and resiliency. Once an alliance forms, positive outcomes can occur when the helping relationship is genuine and perceived as helpful by the helper and the one being helped, the traumatized individual has some hope, and the interaction in the helping relationship stimulates a healthy change (Gelso, 2014).

In *Alice's Adventures in Wonderland*, the caucus race symbolizes the Dodo effect, or how common factors are beneficial. In Carroll's novel, a running race begins with all participants, including Alice, and ends when the Dodo proclaims, "Everybody has won, and all must have prizes" (1865, p. 34). This positive result is good news for everyone. Such a good ending is a common factor in all therapies. Providing sincere support to someone in crisis is helpful. The affirming relationship between you and the person with trauma is essential (Wampold, 2015). According to researchers, these common factors, including the relationship between the helper and the person needing support, contribute up to 49.6% of the positive outcomes for the person (Cuijpers et al., 2012). This study aligns with a previous one that showed that 30% of the positive effects relate to common factors (Lambert, 1992). We emphasize to novice counselors that providing a safe environment with a safe person is powerful.

Treating Trauma

While social support helps many, some people need professional help: pharmaco-therapy or psychotherapy. Multiple studies have aimed to find the most effective treatment for intervention in trauma-related stress. Typically, trauma-focused approaches are the first line of treatment as those address traumatic memories, avoidance, hyperarousal symptoms, and the cognitive imbalance that is a conse-quence of trauma exposure (Watkins et al., 2018). There are non-trauma-focused treatments available that may reduce posttraumatic stress symptoms. However, some are without significant evidence to warrant their use unless a clinician determines they are appropriate for specific clients. Professionals who work with trauma victims achieve the best results when they combine their clinical expertise with the best available external evidence (Sackett et al., 1996). The use of established guidelines for treatment is of utmost importance.

Established Guidelines for Treatment of Adults

Wise professionals stay attuned to current practices and guidelines in helping anyone with trauma stress. However, some clinicians are hesitant to use these strategies for several reasons. There tends to be a perception that using such approaches requires too much time to learn. Some therapists note that conflicting guidelines and pro-cedures may not apply to clients with comorbid conditions. Other reasons include the belief that the best care is what the practitioner has successfully used before and that manualized treatment parameters are inflexible (Martin et al., 2021). While these barriers may be partially true, it is essential to understand the purpose of such recommendations. Guidelines are not mandates or requirements. Instead, they are recommendations based on a large body of evidence (Watkins et al., 2018). Due to the inattention to providing evidence-based care, the risk of developing PTSD rises. This finding occurs across socioeconomic status and culture. Insufficient training, supervi-sion, and fear of re-traumatizing clients play an additional role (Forbes et al., 2020). While intervention efficacy must be present, that alone is insufficient in determining best practices. Instead, the combination of this evidence and clinical expertise is vital in treatment planning (Sackett et al., 1996).

For those clinicians offering counseling services, evidence-based care is optimal, and several high-quality reviews are provided by the American Psychological Association, the International Society for Traumatic Stress Studies (ISTSS), the National Institute for Health and Care Excellence (NICE), and the U.S. Department of Veterans Affairs and Department of Defense (VA/DoD). Each organization provides recommendations based on a review or grading system (Forbes et al., 2020). The review committees offer guidelines grounded upon one or more of the following: treatment efficacy, evidence strength, balance for health or harm, patient preferences, applicability to populations, patient or provider values, equity, acceptability, and feasibility (Bisson et al., 2020; VA/DoD Clinical Practice Guideline Working Group, 2023; Watkins et al., 2018).

There are many options for the treatment of Acute Stress Disorder, PTSD, and post-traumatic stress symptoms. One must remember that a lack of evidence does not necessarily mean a treatment is ineffective. It may mean, for example, there are not yet enough studies to determine the level of efficacy (Bisson et al., 2020). The recommendations for early interventions aim at providing care for someone with traumatic stress symptoms or who meets the criteria for Acute Stress Disorder within the first three months after the traumatic event. Table 6.1 lists the treatment recommendations for early intervention. It is not possible to discuss all the recommendations within this text; however, the most highly recommended approaches, Cognitive Behavioral Therapy (CBT), Cognitive Processing Therapy (CPT), Prolonged Exposure therapy (PE), and Eye Movement and Desensitization Reprocessing (EMDR), will be explored further.

While these treatments are recommended for early intervention, there are similar but separate recommendations for intervention three months after the traumatic experience. While similar, additional approaches have been studied for psychotherapy. Table 6.2: Recommendations for Intervention after the First Three Months lists these recommendations.

TABLE 6.1 Recommendations for Early Intervention within the First Three Months

Agency	Early Interventions (Acute Stress Disorder)
	Standard Recommendation
ISTSS	[1]CBT-T, [3]CT, [4]EMDR
	Interventions with Emerging Evidence
ISTSS	Internet-based guided self-help; structured writing interventions
	Insufficient Evidence to Recommend
ISTSS	Behavioral activation, brief [2]CPT, Internet virtual reality therapy, nurse-led psychological intervention, supportive counseling, telephone-based [1]CBT-T

Source: Bisson et al. (2020).
Note: [1]Cognitive Behavior Therapy with a trauma focus; [2]Cognitive Processing Therapy; [3]Cognitive Therapy; [4]Eye Movement and Desensitization and Reprocessing.

Established Guidelines for Treatment of Adults

TABLE 6.2 Recommendations for Intervention after the First Three Months

Agency	Interventions (PTSD)
Strongly Recommend	
APA	*CBT, [2]CPT, PE, [3]CT
ISTSS	[2]CPT, CT, [4]EMDR, Individual [1]CBT-T, [5]PE
NICE	[1]CBT-T
VA/DoD	[6]BEP, [2]CPT, [4]EMDR, NET, [5]PE, Written Exposure Therapy
Recommend	
APA	[6]BEP, [4]EMDR, [7]NET
ISTSS	*CBT without trauma focus, group [1]CBT-T, guided Internet-based *CBT, NET, Present-centered therapy
VA/DoD	[8]SIT; [9]PCT, [10]IPT
WHO	*CBT; [4]EMDR
Emerging Evidence	
ISTSS	Couples [1]CBT-T, group and individual [1]CBT-T, single-session *CBT, virtual reality therapy, Written exposure therapy
Insufficient Evidence to Recommend	
ISTSS	[6]BEP, Dialogical exposure therapy, emotion freedom techniques, group interpersonal therapy, individual psychotherapy/self-help, interpersonal psychotherapy, psychodynamic psychotherapy, psychoeducation, supportive counseling, trauma-focused counseling

Source: American Psychological Association (2017), Bisson et al. (2020), Forbes et al. (2020), Martin et al. (2021), VA/DoD (2017), and VA/DoD (2023).
Note: *Cognitive Behavior Therapy; [1]Cognitive Behavior Therapy with trauma focus; [2]Cognitive Processing Therapy; [3]Cognitive Therapy; [4]Eye Movement & Desensitization Reprocessing; [5]Prolonged Exposure Therapy; [6]Brief Eclectic Psychotherapy; [7]Narrative Exposure Therapy; [8]Stress Inoculation Training; [9]Person-Centered Therapy; [10]Interpersonal Psychotherapy.

Evidence-Based Treatments for Adults

There is agreement among these researchers and concerned organizations about the best treatments for PTSD in adults. However, these do not encompass all therapeutic approaches to trauma therapy, nor does this diminish the possible efficacy of other methods. For most, the following treatments are considered the first line of treatment for adults with PTSD. These include Cognitive Behavioral Therapy with a trauma focus, Cognitive Processing Therapy, Prolonged Exposure therapy, and EMDR.

Cognitive Behavioral Therapy-Trauma-Focused

Cognitive Behavioral Therapy with a trauma focus (CBT-T) is the first line of treatment for PTSD (Bisson et al., 2020; Martin et al., 2021). The goal of CBT-T focuses on the client's traumatic stress and addresses the negative cognitions and intrusive thoughts or memories that surface with the arousal symptoms. Typically, sessions include psychoeducation, relaxation, stress management, affect regulation, cognitive restructuring, exposure work to process traumatic memories, and homework assignments (Bisson et al., 2020). CBT-T is helpful for adults, adolescents, and children. CBT-T may be offered in individual, family caregiver, or group modalities through face-to-face sessions or online (Forbes et al., 2020).

People with PTSD often have intense negative thoughts about the trauma and find it difficult to process in a broader context. They also have powerful memories and associations with the trauma, which can cause them to relive it involuntarily (Ehlers & Clark, 2000). As a result, people develop strategies that hinder their ability to function in daily life. They might display shame and guilt along with the traumatic memory (Kubany et al., 2004). Due to negative evaluations and heightened arousal, they may avoid people, places, things, or other stimuli that rouse adverse reactions (Cusack et al., 2016).

CBT-T uses behavioral techniques and cognitive restructuring to help clients change their thoughts and beliefs. The treatment includes sharing the trauma story either verbally or in written form. There are concerns about trauma-focused treatment possibly causing more distress or adverse side effects (Cusack et al., 2016). However, there is little evidence that those concerns are associated with CBT-T (APA, 2017; VA/DoD, 2023). One form of CBT-T is the Trauma-Focused Cognitive-Behavioral Therapy (TF-CBT) approach. Lee and Bowles (2020) recommend using it with adolescents and children, although practitioners can use it with any age group. Other CBT-T approaches include Dialectical Behavior Therapy (DBT), telephone-based CBT-T, and brief CBT-T. Additional treatments include CBT in the framework, such as CPT, EMDR, NET, and PE, which are discussed separately (Lee & Bowles, 2020).

CBT-T approaches should be based on validated manuals, occur over a minimum of eight sessions, and include information about trauma reactions, strategies for managing arousal and flashbacks, and safety planning. The course of treatment should incorporate a stabilization phase, trauma processing, integration and consolidation, and continued monitoring or follow-up (NICE, 2018).

Is CBT-T better than other approaches? This question is interesting, and the response varies from study to study. EMDR was slightly more effective than CBT in reducing intrusion and hyperarousal symptoms, according to a meta-analysis. However, there was no significant difference between the two approaches in reducing avoidance symptoms (Lee et al., 2016). Another study showed that trauma-focused therapy is more effective than non-trauma-focused approaches for PTSD (Chen et al., 2015). One meta-analysis noted small effect sizes favoring EMDR for reducing depressive symptoms, but the long-term effects were not found to be more favorable than CBT (Cuijpers et al., 2020). Other researchers report that CBT, EMDR, and PE are the most effective, but none are better than the other (Bisson et al., 2020; Erford et al., 2016; Lenz et al., 2017; Sloan et al., 2013). Consider the following case.

Nurture Understanding

Sally was a 32-year-old divorced female with three children ages 6, 8, and 12. Two of the children, females, had auditory processing disorders. Sally's history included sexual abuse as a child, sexual assault as an adult, and domestic violence. The psychiatrist diagnosed Sally with PTSD, Major Depressive Disorder, and borderline personality disorder. Before she engaged with her new therapist, Sally's hospitalizations due to suicidal ideation and gestures totaled 16 times within four years. The ongoing suicidal crisis and other therapy-interfering behaviors like parasuicidal behavior, manipulation, and boundary violation hindered Sally's progress. The new therapist, Amanda, thought trauma-focused CBT might be a good option with Sally.

- In what ways would CBT-T be a good option for Sally?
- What must the therapist consider when choosing an approach for a client like Sally?
- What other approaches might be better for Sally? Why?

Cognitive Processing Therapy

Cognitive Processing Therapy (CPT) focuses on evaluating and modifying problematic cognitions that develop after the trauma (Bisson et al., 2020). While CPT is a CBT-T approach, it is considered separately due to its intentional protocol which varies from other CBT-T models. CPT uses social cognitive and informed emotional processing theories (Resick et al., 2012). In this approach, the assumption is that survivors attempt to make sense of the trauma, which may lead to distorted cognitions regarding themselves, others, or the world around them. In their attempt to integrate this tragic event, people may assimilate, accommodate, or over-accommodate. Assimilation occurs when incoming stimuli are changed to confirm beliefs typically based on shame and guilt (Watkins et al., 2018). For example, a person may say, "My unit was killed when they drove over the IED (improvised explosive device) because I was not there to spot it." Over-accommodation occurs when one's beliefs are altered to prevent such an event from occurring again (Resick et al., 2012). One example might be, "Because this happened, I am untrustworthy or do not deserve respect."

The core ingredients of CPT include psychoeducation, Socratic dialogue, cognitive worksheets, affirmations, addressing cognitive avoidance, and providing noncontingent activities for oneself or those that are not earned but freely given for being human (Olff et al., 2020). CPT aims at activation of cognitive memory by writing the index event and exploring the beliefs resulting from assimilation and over-accommodation. Typically, clients become fixed on issues related to safety, trust, power and control, esteem, and intimacy (Thomas et al., 2023). CPT is a manualized, time-limited treatment occurring over 12 sessions that uses cognitive restructuring and emotional processing (Thomas et al., 2023). Exposure elements aid clients in healthy accommodation as the client considers why the trauma occurred and how it has changed their belief system (Resick et al., 2012).

How effective is CPT? Meta-analyses suggest that CPT is effective in reducing PTSD symptoms (Cusack et al., 2016). In addition, the rates of participants who no longer met the criteria for PTSD ranged from 30 to 97%. Approximately 51% of participants who received CPT lost the PTSD diagnosis, which was more favorable than participants who were on a waitlist, reviewed a self-help book, or other treatments as usual (Jonas et al., 2013). CPT is concerned about the schema or themes surrounding the traumatic event, not just the possible distorted thoughts surrounding trauma.

Cultivate Knowledge

Cognitive Processing Therapy aims at changing the ineffective default themes surrounding safety, trust, power and control, esteem, and intimacy. Think about someone you have helped that had PTSD or C-PTSD. Answer the following questions:

- What struggles did this person have with feeling safe?
- In what ways did they have difficulty trusting you or the care you provided?
- What problems occurred surrounding power and control?
- How did the person view themselves? What issues did they have with self-esteem?
- How did trauma affect their relationships?

Established Guidelines for Treatment of Adults

Prolonged Exposure Therapy

Prolonged Exposure Therapy is based on emotional processing theory and suggests that trauma is not processed emotionally at the time of occurrence (Watkins et al., 2018). The theory suggests that trauma is stored as cognitive representations, feared stimuli, fear responses, and connections to the stimuli. According to Foa et al. (2007), these fear structures are unhealthy when a trauma victim responds with fear to daily occurrences that are innocuous. Prolonged Exposure Therapy focuses on changing these fear structures. Two processes are involved: fear response activation and new evidence of rational information that conflicts with erroneous beliefs in the fear structure (Foa et al., 2007).

In between 8 and 15 sessions, clients receive psychoeducation, self-regulation skills training, and exposure, including imaginal and in vivo exposures and postexposure processing (Olff et al., 2020). The imaginal exposure encourages the client to approach memories, thoughts, and emotions surrounding the index event that is typically avoided. They rehearse the narrative repeatedly, tape recording it, and replay it at home for further exposure (Foa et al., 2007).

In a meta-analysis on effective treatments for PTSD, patients receiving PE had better outcomes than 85% of the control patients at the end of treatment (Powers et al., 2010). Among those participants, 41–95% lost their PTSD diagnosis by the end of treatment (Jonas et al., 2013). In two recent meta-analyses, PE evidence of strength was as high as, if not higher than, other psychological intervention protocols for PTSD (Forman-Hoffman et al., 2018; Schnurr et al., 2022).

Eye Movement & Desensitization Reprocessing (EMDR)

Eye Movement & Desensitization Reprocessing is a brief psychotherapy that has three primary foci, including memories, present disturbances, and future actions with a standardized, eight-phase protocol using bilateral physical stimulation with eye movements, taps, or tones, affect regulation skills, positive belief, desensitization, body scan, and future processing (Olff et al., 2020). The client processes targeted trauma memories, the associated thoughts, emotional responses, and bodily sensations. Some clinicians theorize that EMDR stimulates an individual's information processing system. The therapist uses limited questioning related to cognitions paired with bilateral stimulation to unblock the client's processing (Bisson et al., 2020). EMDR is included as a first-line treatment recommendation for many organizations (Martin et al., 2021). Francine Shapiro developed the procedure in the late 1980s based on her observations that trauma memories lessened with eye movements. However, the mechanism through which this occurs is still being determined. Some researchers believe cognitive behavioral elements are responsible for positive outcomes, not eye movements. Others suggest that eye movements contribute to the positive effects (Cuijpers et al., 2020).

Research on EMDR has grown since the first clinical trials in 1994, with mixed results. Cuijpers et al. (2020) reported a small effect size post-treatment and at maintenance, while other meta-analyses reported moderate to large effect sizes (Chen et al., 2015; Cusack et al., 2016). However, some studies did not include a population diagnosed with PTSD, and others did not have sufficient methodological quality (Rasines-Laudes & Serrano-Pintado, 2023). The long-term effects of EMDR are unknown, and the results are controversial (Cuijpers et al., 2020). One problem noted was the number of studies with high-risk bias versus those with low-risk bias. In other words, the researchers' bias may have influenced the outcomes (Cuijpers et al., 2020). There are other problems with research on EMDR, including the few number of studies with low-risk bias, little significant difference between EMDR and other therapies, considerable indication of researcher allegiance to the protocol, and insufficient evidence of efficacy (Lee et al., 2016; Schubert et al., 2010; van den Hout et al., 2011). However, the popularity of the treatment method remains and is a highly recommended treatment approach for PTSD.

This discussion examined the four most highly recommended approaches for trauma treatment: CBT, CPT, PE, and EMDR. Each of these treatment approaches, as well as other trauma methods, include the following components (Figure 6.1):

- Stabilization and grounding
- Therapeutic alliance
- Trauma narrative and processing
- Cognitive restructuring.

Several other approaches are worthy of consideration, including Narrative Exposure Therapy, which combines components from CBT and PE, and Brief Eclectic Psychotherapy, which combines CBT, imaginal exposure, and grief therapy. Emerging and promising therapies are available, and we recommend you continually check on those as research clinical trials support their use.

Established Guidelines for Treatment of Adults

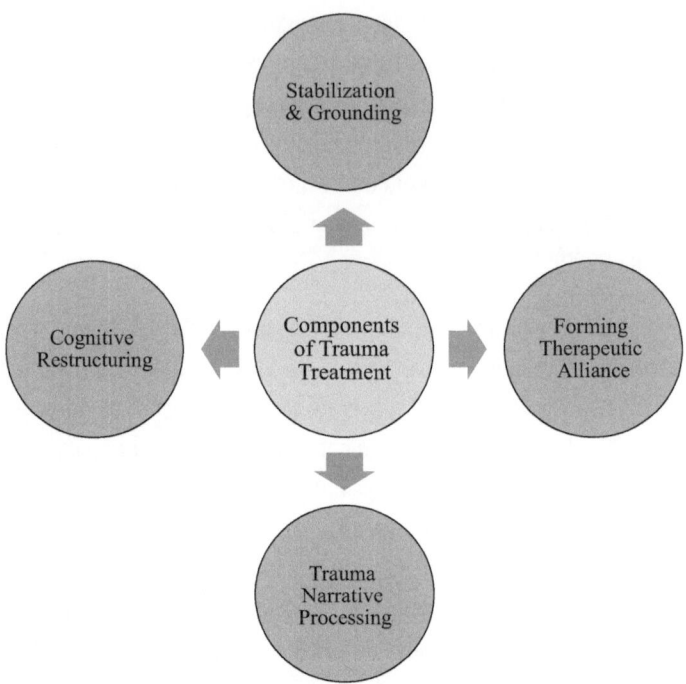

FIGURE 6.1   Components of Trauma Treatment.

Tending Your Technique

Mark is an African American, married, and a police officer in his mid-thirties. He has three small children. His dream as a child was to be an officer serving his community. Mark grew up in a poverty-stricken community that was unsafe. He witnessed domestic violence, experienced childhood sexual assault by his stepfather, and was exposed to violent deaths due to gang-related activity in his neighborhood. Two years ago, Mark was called to the scene of a shooting where he tried to rescue the children. Of the six children in the house, three were dead, and three were seriously injured and life-flighted to hospitals. He was overwhelmed by the scene and found himself frozen at one point. Afterward, Mark experienced PTSD symptoms and began drinking heavily. He has been unable to work since the event and was referred for PE therapy:

- What aspects of Prolonged Exposure Therapy might be beneficial for Mark?
- What would be different about this PE therapy compared to CPT?
- In what ways would EMDR be a better approach for Mark?

Recommendations for Treatment of Children & Youth

Treatment of trauma in youth requires considering the influence of parenting and caregivers' reactions. The caregiver's functioning level and how they care for the child is critical. Research suggests that sensitive and attentive care during or following a trauma can mediate the effects of trauma on a child's functioning. However, if a caregiver is punitive, detached, or neglectful, this parenting style can worsen the effects of trauma on youth (McLaughlin & Lambert, 2018; Osofsky & Osofsky, 2018). Since 65% of children encounter at least one traumatic event by age 16, child-serving systems must recognize that trauma, abuse, and neglect have a lasting impact on brain function (Bartlett, 2020). Trauma-informed care for youth must be comprehensive and offer multiple avenues of support. Children and youth fare better after trauma when care is consistent and caring and offers safety and predictability (Bartlett et al., 2017).

Recommendations for trauma treatment in children differ according to developmental stages, availability of caregivers, and ability of caregivers to participate. For children older than seven, individual trauma-focused therapy should include a stabilization phase, a trauma narration and processing phase, an integration and consolidation phase, and a monitoring phase. Regarding children aged 3–6, the recommendations include Child–Parent Psychotherapy (CPP) or Trauma-Focused Cognitive Behavioral Therapy (TF-CBT) for preschoolers. For children under three, CPP is preferred above TF-CBT or Preschool PTSD Psychotherapy (Cohen, 2023). The International Society for Traumatic Stress Studies strongly recommends CBT-T and EMDR for children and youth (Jensen et al., 2020). The American Academy of Child and Adolescent Psychiatry recommends trauma-focused psychotherapies as the primary front-line treatment. If a child or adolescent does not respond to this treatment, EMDR is suggested (Lucio & Nelson, 2016; NICE, 2018). The efficacy of treatments in children and adolescents varies among studies. A large study showed that TF-CBT had more significant effects on reducing PTSD symptoms than EMDR (Gutermann et al., 2016). Another research review of TF-CBT compared to EMDR for reducing PTSD symptoms in youth found both had a moderate effect (Mavranezouli et al., 2020).

Limited research exists on treating C-PTSD in children and youth (Alisic et al., 2014; Jensen et al., 2020). The International Society of Traumatic Stress Studies states that there is insufficient evidence to support specific treatments for complex PTSD in children and adolescents. It suggests modifications to current treatments for PTSD (ISTSS,

2019). The priority of treating youth with C-PTSD should be to develop emotional and interpersonal regulation skills and bolster self-esteem prior to treating the trauma (Knipschild et al., 2023). Exposure therapy may be helpful, and approaches include PE and Narrative Exposure Therapy (Huang et al., 2022).

Parent Education Approaches

For younger children, parent education approaches may be the best strategies. These can be offered in groups, family, or dyad settings. Several beneficial approaches exist, including the Child Adult Relationship Enhancement (CARE) program, Daring to Care, Attachment and Biobehavioral Catch-Up, Child-Parent Psychotherapy (CPP), and Parent–Child Interaction Therapy (PCIT). Each is described briefly.

Child Adult Relationship Enhancement (CARE)

The CARE program is designed for older children, with a modification for preschool children, PriCARE (Gurwitch et al., 2016). CARE is designed to strengthen positive relationships between adults and youth aged 2–18. It uses adult learning principles and live feedback for skill retention (Kaminski et al., 2008). This program helps to improve adult–child relationships, child behaviors, and caregiver confidence and decreases corporal punishment (Messer et al., 2018; Schilling et al., 2016).

Daring to Care

The Daring to Care approach, developed in Finland, focuses on parents with a trauma history. The program recognizes parents' difficulties in being available, nurturing, and effectively disciplining their children (Beeghly & Tronick, 2011). This approach also recognizes the parent's difficulties in mentalization, which affects the caregiver's ability to respond in healthy ways to the child (Fonagy et al., 2007). Daring to Care developed from the recommendations of ISTSS for a group recovery model to provide psychoeducation about trauma symptoms and emotion regulation skills for parents to help them become better skilled at parenting, mainly when triggered or during dissociation (Reddemann & Piedfort-Marin, 2017; Steele et al., 2017). Two versions of this approach exist, one with 24 sessions and another with 13 sessions. The program combines cognitive and trauma-focused techniques with attachment and mentalization approaches. This program is open to parents who live with or co-parent children and can reflect on how their trauma affects their parenting. The closed group accommodates 6–8 parents. Participants must not have active substance use problems or be in crisis (Friberg et al., 2019).

Attachment and Biobehavioral Catch-Up

A third approach that addresses the parent-child relationship is the Attachment and Biobehavioral Catch-Up (ABC) program, a ten 10-session home visitation program designed for mothers and infants up to age 2. This manualized intervention has three primary foci: nurturing a distressed infant, following the infant's lead when not distressed, and avoiding harsh or frightening behavior (Lyons-Ruth & Jacobvitz, 2016). The first goal is to aid parents in responding to nurturing when the child is unable or does not start such and is in distress or when behaving in a nurturing way is unnatural for the parent. The subsequent goals assist the parent in learning how to respond to the infant during non-distress and offer a safe environment. This approach increases parental sensitivity and decreases negative responses (O'Byrne et al., 2023; Roben et al., 2017). The efficacy of this approach shows fewer children with disorganized attachment, decreases in cortisol levels, more normal autonomic nervous system responses, and improved neural activity and brain functioning (Bernard et al., 2012; Garnett et al., 2020; Tabachnick et al., 2019; Valadez et al., 2020).

Child–Parent Psychotherapy (CPP)

The most recommended approach for young children under five years old is Child–Parent Psychotherapy (CPP). This approach addresses the emotional and behavioral issues common in children with trauma. The goal is to restore trust and safety and affect regulation (Lieberman et al., 2015). CPP reduces PTSD symptoms and behavior problems and has a positive impact on caregivers. This approach is most effective for families with chronic trauma. However, CPP is not recommended if the child and caregiver do not have consistent and ongoing contact or if the parent has a mental health condition that includes hallucinations (Lucio & Nelson, 2016).

Parent–Child Interaction Therapy (PCIT)

Parent–Child Interaction Therapy (PCIT) is recommended for children aged 2–17 and their caregivers. The approach employs a dyadic intervention involving parent and

Recommendations for Treatment of Children & Youth

child using attachment theory, behavior management, play therapy, and social learning theory. Treatment comprises two phases: Child-directed interaction and parent-directed interaction. Each phase consists of 6–10 sessions using assessment, *in vivo* coaching, and live feedback (Funderburk & Eyberg, 2011). The goal is strengthening the parent–child relationship through PRIDE skills: praise of appropriate behaviors, reflections of appropriate speech and active listening, imitation of appropriate behavior, descriptions focused on the child's play and providing attention, and enjoying the relationship (Gurwitch et al., 2017). The focus is consistency, predictability, and parental follow-through (Masud et al., 2019).

This discussion of therapeutic interventions and parent interaction approaches is incomplete. Other meaningful and helpful programs are available to assist those working with children and adolescents. Further research is needed to determine the efficacy of these approaches with C-PTSD.

Gather Self-Awareness

Several approaches for children and adolescents were described. As you reflect on this, or if you know of other treatment types, think about the following:

- Which of the approaches mentioned sounds most appealing to you and fits your understanding of trauma and children?
- Have you heard of other evidence-based treatments? What are your thoughts about these?

A Flourishing Focus

When we think about the treatment of trauma in adults, children, and adolescents, we desire to pay tribute to the individual and find ways to dignify their journey. The goal is not to return a person to a pre-trauma state but rather to bring them to a new state of physical and psychological health. The salutogenic approach helps us by focusing on how responses to trauma stressors can strengthen a person's sense of coherence, self-efficacy, and well-being (Mittelmark & Bauer, 2022). This understanding of treatment moves from viewing trauma as a pathogen attacking a person's system and something that must be reduced or erased to a recognition of how posttrauma recovery fortifies human beings. In a recent discussion with licensure candidates, we spoke of the Japanese philosophy and art of kintsugi. Broken pottery pieces are reunited in the art form using gold-laced epoxy seams. Interestingly, this mending produces beautiful work and strengthens the original vessel, thus making it more valuable (Buetow & Wallis, 2019). To clarify our position, it is not the adverse experience that produces such creative development but the innate capacities of individuals for growth. Life invariably brings terrible circumstances, and human beings possess stunning abilities to transcend those struggles.

An infant is born and soon develops a sense of coherence. As the infant develops, growth occurs intrapsychic as they achieve milestones, create a sense of self, and form attachments. The child's sense of coherence increases as they interact in sociocultural and historical contexts and find external resources that provide support (Mittelmark & Bauer, 2022). Life experiences bring challenges and new insights, allowing the maturing human to generate further resistance resources such as practical knowledge and a sense of control over their responses to experiences. As young adults launch into careers and long-term relationships, they become perceptive, flexible, and rational. Flourishing occurs as they face life experiences that are consistent and manageable, and they participate in shaping the outcome (Mittelmark & Bauer, 2022). However, for some, the unforeseeable strikes, and life appears to collapse. For others, they enter the world without the advantage of a secure environment. Still, others find they cannot control everything, learning that some things transpire that are painful and uncontrollable. For these people, therapy becomes a curative place.

The goal of treatment for trauma from a resilience perspective is providing safety, a place for the client to speak the truth, and strengthening the person, like a kintsugi art piece. Therapy means focusing on the person, their story, and how that shapes their purpose in life. Having a client redefine who they are post-trauma becomes critical, rather than having them identify themselves as a diagnosis. Clients do not come to us broken but as creative, resourceful, and whole human beings needing transformation. In counseling, we move from "I am bulimic," "I am an alcoholic," or "I am a victim of child abuse" to "I am a person who struggles with bulimia, substance addiction, or traumatic symptoms, and one who is rising above those to become a person with purpose." This way, clients develop a constructive narrative that complements and strengthens their identity. The metamorphosis task promotes the individual's sense of coherence, supporting their understanding, helping them identify inner and external resources, supporting their search for meaning, and discovering their adaptive capacities (Langeland & Vinje, 2022). These goals and tasks can be incorporated into

A Flourishing Focus

evidence-based treatment approaches for adults, children, and adolescents, ultimately increasing their subjective well-being (Dube & Rishi, 2017). This is truly the best part of working with survivors.

Chapter Summary

This chapter discussed evidence-based treatments for trauma, focusing on trauma-informed care, trauma-specific services, and trauma-informed practice. It emphasized the importance of understanding the impact of trauma on individuals' lives and the need for trauma-informed care, particularly for those who have experienced painful events. The chapter highlighted the significance of providing valuable support to individuals with trauma, emphasizing the role of social encouragement and the impact of social support in reducing adverse mental health outcomes and enhancing recovery.

In addition, the chapter summarized various parent education approaches for children who have experienced trauma, including the Child Adult Relationship Enhancement (CARE) program, Daring to Care, Attachment and Biobehavioral Catch-Up, Child–Parent Psychotherapy (CPP), and Parent–Child Interaction Therapy (PCIT). Each approach was described, emphasizing the importance of sensitive and attentive care during or following trauma as a protective factor for children's functioning.

Furthermore, it offered the most recommended evidence-based psychotherapy treatments for trauma, such as Cognitive Behavioral Therapy (CBT), Cognitive Processing Therapy (CPT), Prolonged Exposure therapy (PE), and Eye Movement and Desensitization Reprocessing (EMDR). The effectiveness of these treatments for trauma was discussed, along with considerations for treating trauma in both adults and children. The chapter addressed the importance of resilience and a salutogenic approach in trauma treatment. It focused on strengthening individuals' sense of coherence and supporting their understanding, search for meaning, and adaptive capacities.

Overall, the document offered a comprehensive overview of evidence-based treatments for trauma, emphasizing the significance of trauma-informed care, the effectiveness of different psychotherapy treatments, and the importance of resilience and salutogenic approaches in trauma treatment. It also underscored the need for supportive and nurturing environments for individuals, notably children, who have experienced trauma.

Chapter Review

Please respond to the following questions:

1. What are the most recommended evidence-based psychotherapy treatments for trauma in adults? Why are these highly recommended?
2. What treatments are recommended for children? Why are these best?
3. How important is resilience and a salutogenic approach in trauma treatment?
4. How can therapy promote a client's sense of coherence and adaptive capacities?

Key Term Assessment

Review the following terms and try to explain each concept.

- Trauma-Focused CBT
- Cognitive Processing Therapy
- Prolonged Exposure Therapy
- EMDR

Resources

The following resources may be helpful. At the time of this writing, they were accessible through the links provided.

- Cognitive Processing Therapy for Posttraumatic Stress Disorder. This site provides information about CPT, approved providers, resources, and how to obtain certification. https://cptforptsd.com
- *Cognitive Processing Therapy for PTSD: A Comprehensive Manual* by Patricia A. Resick, Candice M. Monson, and Kathleen M. Chard. This is the essential manual for the CPT approach.
- EMDR International Association (EMDRIA). This site is the certifying body for EMDR practice. It provides information, research, resources, approved providers, and training opportunities for those providers who desire to learn the skills for EMDR. https://www.emdria.org
- *Eye Movement Desensitization and Reprocessing (EMDR) Therapy: Basic Principles, Protocols, and Procedures* by Francine Shapiro. This is the essential manual for the EMDR approach.

Chapter Summary

- Prolonged Exposure (PE) for PTSD. This site is sponsored by the National Center for PTSD by the U.S. Department of Veteran Affairs. It briefly overviews PE and suggests using PE Coach, a mobile application. https://www.ptsd.va.gov/understand_tx/prolonged_exposure.asp#:~:text=Prolonged%20Exposure%20(PE)%20is%20a,been%20avoiding%20since%20your%20trauma

- PTSD Consultation Program: Training in Prolonged Exposure. This site is sponsored by the National Center for PTSD by the U.S. Department of Veteran Affairs. It allows licensed mental health providers who treat veterans to receive free in-person training and six months of weekly phone consultation. https://www.ptsd.va.gov/professional/consult/trainings.asp

- *Prolonged Exposure Therapy for PTSD: Emotional Processing of Traumatic Experiences* by Edna Foa, Elizabeth Hembree, and Barbara Olaslov Rothbaum. This is the essential manual and therapist guide for the PE approach.

- PTSD Treatment Decision Aid: The Choice is Yours. This site provides information about PTSD, treatment options, and a decision aid to help clients or patients determine the best treatment route. https://www.ptsd.va.gov/apps/decisionaid/

- *Trauma-Focused CBT for Children and Adolescents: Treatment Applications* by Judith A. Cohen, Anthony P. Mannarino, and Esther Deblinger. This is the essential manual for TF-CBT.

- Trauma-Focused Cognitive Behavioral Therapy National Therapist Certification Program. This site provides information about TF-CBT, approved certified therapists, resources, and how to obtain certification. https://tfcbt.org

References

Alisic, E., Zalta, A. K., van Wesel, F., Larsen, S. E., Hafstad, G. S., Hassanpour, K., & Smid, G. E. (2014). Rates of post-traumatic stress disorder in trauma-exposed children and adolescents: Meta-analysis. *The British Journal of Psychiatry: The Journal of Mental Science, 204*, 335–340. https://doi.org/10.1192/bjp.bp.113.131227

American Psychiatric Association (APA). (2017). *Clinical practice guidelines for the treatment of PTSD*. American Psychiatric Association. https://www.apa.org/ptsd-guideline/ptsd.pdf

American Psychiatric Association (APA). (2022). *Diagnostic and statistical manual of mental disorders* (5th ed.) American Psychiatric Association.

Bartlett, J. D. (2020). Screening for childhood adversity: Contemporary challenges and recommendations. *Adversity and Resilience Science*, *1*, 65–79. https://doi.org/10.1007/s42844-020-00004-8

Bartlett, J. D., Smith, S., & Bringewatt, E. (2017). Helping young children who have experienced trauma: Policies and strategies for early care and education. *Child Trends*. https://www.childtrends.org/wp-content/uploads/2017/04/2017-19ECETrauma.pdf

Beeghly, M., & Tronick, E. (2011). Early resilience in the context of parent-infant relationships: A social developmental perspective. *Current Problems in Pediatric and Adolescent Health Care*, *41*(7), 197–201. https://doi.org/10.1016/j.cppeds.2011.02.005

Bernard, K., Dozier, M., Bick, J., Lewis-Morrarty, E., Lindhiem, O., & Carlson, E. (2012). Enhancing attachment organization among maltreated children: Results of a randomized clinical trial. *Child Development*, *83*(2), 623–636. https://doi.org/10.1111/j.1467-8624.2011.01712.x

Bisson, J. I., Lewis, C., & Roberts, N. P. (2020). ISTSS PTSD prevention and treatment guidelines: Methodology. In D. Forbes, J. I. Bisson, C. M. Monson, & L. Berliner (Eds.), *Effective treatments for PTSD: Practice guidelines from the International Society for Traumatic Stress Studies* (pp. 90–108). The Guilford Press.

Buetow, S., & Wallis, K. (2019). The beauty in perfect imperfection. *Journal of Medical Humanities*, *40*, 389–394. https://doi.org/10.1007/s10912-017-9500-2

Carroll, L. (1865). *Alice's adventures in wonderland*. Macmillan.

Chen, L., Zhang, G., Hu, M., & Liang, X. (2015). Eye movement desensitization and reprocessing versus cognitive-behavioral therapy for adult posttraumatic stress disorder: Systematic review and meta-analysis. *The Journal of Nervous and Mental Disease*, *203*(6), 443–451. https://doi.org/10.1097/NMD.0000000000000306

Cohen, J. A. (2023). *Posttraumatic stress disorder in children and adolescents: Trauma-focused psychotherapy*. Wolters Kluwer.

Cuijpers, P., Driessen, E., Hollon, S. D., van Oppen, P., Barth, J., & Andersson, G. (2012). The efficacy of non-directive supportive therapy for adult depression: A meta-analysis. *Clinical Psychology Review*, *32*(4), 280–291. https://doi.org/10.1016/j.cpr.2012.01.003

Cuijpers, P., van Veen, S. C., Sijbrandij, M., Yoder, W., & Cristea, I. A. (2020). Eye movement desensitization and reprocessing for mental health problems? A systematic review and meta-analysis. *Cognitive Behaviour Therapy*, *49*(3), 165–180. https://doi.org/10.1080/16506073.2019.1703801

Cusack, K., Jonas, D. E., Forneris, C. A., Wines, C., Sonis, J., Middleton, J. C., Feltner, C., Brownley, K. A., Olmsted, K. R., Greenblatt, A., Weil, A., & Gaynes, B. N. (2016). Psychological treatments for adults with posttraumatic stress disorder: A systematic review and meta-analysis. *Clinical Psychology Review*, *43*, 128–141. https://doi.org/10.1016/j.cpr.2015.10.003

Danielson, C. K., Cohen, J. R., Adams, Z. W., Youngstrom, E. A., Soltis, K., Amstadter, A. B., & Ruggiero, K. J. (2017). Clinical decision-making following disasters: Efficient identification of PTSD risk in adolescents. *Journal of Abnormal Child Psychology, 45*(1), 117–119. https://doi.org/10.1007/s10802-016-0159-3

Dube, S. R., & Rishi, S. (2017). Utilizing the salutogenic paradigm to investigate well-being among adult survivors of childhood sexual abuse and other adversities. *Child Abuse & Neglect, 66,* 130–141. https://doi.org/10.1016/j.chiabu.2017.01.026

Dückers, M. L. A. (2017). A multilayered psychosocial resilience framework and its implications for community-focused crisis management. *Journal of Contingencies and Crisis Management, 25*(3), 182–187. https://doi.org/10.1111/1468-5973.12183

Ehlers, A., & Clark, D. M. (2000). A cognitive model of posttraumatic stress disorder. *Behaviour Research and Therapy, 38*(4), 319–345. https://doi.org/10.1016/s0005-7967(99)00123-0

Erford, B. T., Gunther, C., Duncan, K., Bardhoshi, G., Dummett, B., Kraft, J., Deferio, K., Falco, M., & Ross, M. (2016). Meta-analysis of counseling outcomes for the treatment of posttraumatic stress disorder. *Journal of Counseling & Development, 94*(1), 13–30. https://doi.org/10.1002/jcad.12058

Foa, E. B., Hembree, E. A., & Rothbaum, B. O. (2007). *Prolonged exposure therapy for PTSD: Emotional processing of traumatic experiences: Therapist guide.* Oxford University Press.

Fonagy, P., Gergely, G., & Target, M. (2007). The parent-infant dyad and the construction of the subjective self. *Journal of Child Psychology and Psychiatry and Allied Disciplines, 48*(3–4), 288–328. https://doi.org/10.1111/j.1469-7610.2007.01727.x

Forbes, D., Bisson, J. I., Monson, C. M., & Berliner, L. (2020). *Effective treatments for PTSD: Practice guidelines from the International Society for Traumatic Stress Studies.* The Guilford Press.

Forman-Hoffman, V., Middleton, J. C., Feltner, C., Gaynes, B. N., Weber, R. P., Bann, C., Viswanathan, M., Lohr, K. N., Baker, C., & Green, J. (2018). Psychological and pharmacological treatments for adults with posttraumatic stress disorder: A systematic review update. *Comparative effectiveness review* (Vol. 207). Agency for Healthcare Research and Quality. https://www.ncbi.nlm.nih.gov/books/NBK525132/

Fredette, C., El-Baalbaki, G., Palardy, V., Rizkallah, E., & Guay, S. (2016). Social support and cognitive–behavioral therapy for posttraumatic stress disorder: A systematic review. *Traumatology, 22*(2), 131–144. https://doi.org/10.1037/trm0000070

Friberg, L., Granö, N., Suokas, A., & Ruismäki, M. (2019). *Parenting difficulties of mothers with childhood trauma: The Daring to Care group intervention pilot study.* University of Helsinki. https://www.researchgate.net/publication/336944976_Parenting_difficulties_of_mothers_with_childhood_trauma_-The_Daring_to_Care_group_intervention_pilot_study

Funderburk, B. W., & Eyberg, S. (2011). Parent–child interaction therapy. In J. C. Norcross, G. R. VandenBos, & D. K. Freedheim (Eds.), *History of psychotherapy: Continuity and change* (2nd ed., pp. 415–420). American Psychological Association. https://doi.org/10.1037/12353-021

Garnett, M., Bernard, K., Hoye, J., Zajac, L., & Dozier, M. (2020). Parental sensitivity mediates the sustained effect of attachment and biobehavioral catch-up on cortisol in middle childhood: A randomized clinical trial. *Psychoneuroendocrinology, 121*, 104809. https://doi.org/10.1016/j.psyneuen.2020.104809

Gelso, C. (2014). A tripartite model of the therapeutic relationship: Theory, research, and practice. *Psychotherapy Research, 24*(2), 117–131. https://doi.org/10.1080/10503307.2013.845920

Gurwitch, R. H., Messer, E. P., & Funderburk, B. W. (2017). Parent–child interaction therapy. In M. A. Landolt, M. Cloitre, & U. Schnyder (Eds.), *Evidence-based treatments for trauma-related disorders in children and adolescents* (pp. 341–362). Springer International Publishing.

Gurwitch, R. H., Messer, E. P., Masse, J., Olafson, E., Boat, B. W., & Putnam, F. W. (2016). Child–Adult Relationship Enhancement (CARE): An evidence-informed program for children with a history of trauma and other behavioral challenges. *Child Abuse & Neglect, 53*, 138–145. https://doi.org/10.1016/j.chiabu.2015.10.016

Gutermann, J., Schreiber, F., Matulis, S., Schwartzkopff, L., Deppe, J., & Steil, R. (2016). Psychological treatments for symptoms of posttraumatic stress disorder in children, adolescents, and young adults: A meta-analysis. *Clinical Child and Family Psychology Review, 19*(2), 77–93. https://doi.org/10.1007/s10567-016-0202-5

Huang, T., Li, H., Tan, S., Xie, S., Cheng, Q., Xiang, Y., & Zhou, X. (2022). The efficacy and acceptability of exposure therapy for the treatment of post-traumatic stress disorder in children and adolescents: A systematic review and meta-analysis. *BMC Psychiatry, 22*, 259. https://doi.org/10.1186/s12888-022-03867-6

Janoff-Bulman, R. (1992). *Shattered assumptions. Towards a new psychology of trauma.* The Free Press.

Jensen, T., Cohen, J., Jaycox, L., & Rosner, R. (2020). Treatment of PTSD and complex PTSD. In Forbes, D., Bisson, J. I., Monson, C. M., & Berliner, L. (Eds.), *Effective treatments for PTSD: Practice guidelines from the International Society for Traumatic Stress Studies* (3rd ed., pp. 385–413). Guilford Press.

Jonas, D. E., Cusack, K., Forneris, C. A., Wilkins, T. M., Sonis, J., Middleton, J. C., Feltner, C., Meredith, D., Cavanaugh, J., Brownley, K. A., Olmsted, K. R., Greenblatt, A., Weil, A., & Gaynes, B. N. (2013). *Psychological and pharmacological treatments for adults with posttraumatic stress disorder (PTSD).* Agency for Healthcare Research and Quality (US).

Kaminski, J. W., Valle, L. A., Filene, J. H., & Boyle, C. L. (2008). A meta-analytic review of components associated with parent training program effectiveness. *Journal of Abnormal Child Psychology, 36*(4), 567–589. https://doi.org/10.1007/s10802-007-9201-9

Kleber, R. J. (2019). Trauma and public mental health: A focused review. *Frontiers in Psychiatry*, *10*, 451. https://doi.org/10.3389/fpsyt.2019.00451

Knipschild, R., Klip, H., van Leeuwaarden, D., van Onna, M. J. R., Lindauer, R. J. L., Staal, W. G., Bicanic, I. A. E., & de Jongh, A. (2023). Treatment of multiple traumatized adolescents by enhancing regulation skills and reducing trauma related symptoms: Rationale, study design, and methods of randomized controlled trial (the Mars-study). *BMC Psychiatry*, *23*, 644. https://doi.org/10.1186/s12888-023-05073-4

Kubany, E. S., Hill, E. E., Owens, J. A., Iannce-Spencer, C., McCaig, M. A., Tremayne, K. J., & Williams, P. L. (2004). Cognitive trauma therapy for battered women with PTSD (CTT-BW). *Journal of Consulting and Clinical Psychology*, *72*(1), 3–18. https://doi.org/10.1023/A:1022019629803

Lambert, M. J. (1992). Psychotherapy outcome research: Implications for integrative and electrical therapists. In J. C. Norcross, & M. R. Goldfield (Eds.), *Handbook of psychotherapy integrations* (pp. 94–129). Basic Books.

Langeland, E., & Vinje, H. F. (2022). Applying salutogenesis in mental healthcare settings. In M. B. Mittelmark, S. Sagy, M. Eriksson, G. Bauer, J. M. Pelikan, B. Lindström, & G. A. Espnes (Eds.), *The handbook of salutogenesis* (pp. 433–439). Springer Open.

Lee, D. J., Schnitzlein, C. W., Wolf, J. P., Vythilingam, M., Rasmusson, A. M., & Hoge, C. W. (2016). Psychotherapy versus pharmacotherapy for posttraumatic stress disorder: Systemic review and meta-analyses to determine first-line treatments. *Depression and Anxiety*, *33*(9), 792–806. https://doi.org/10.1002/da.22511

Lee, E., & Bowles, K. (2020). Navigating treatment recommendations for PTSD: A rapid review. *International Journal of Mental Health*, *52*(1), 4–44. https://doi.org/10.1080/00207411.2020.1781407

Lenz, A. S., Haktanir, A., & Callender, K. (2017). Meta-analysis of trauma-focused therapies for treating the symptoms of posttraumatic stress disorder. *Journal of Counseling & Development*, *95*(3), 339–353. https://doi.org/10.1002/jcad.12148

Lieberman, A. F., Ghosh Ippen, C., & Van Horn, P. (2015). *Don't hit my mommy: A manual for child-parent psychotherapy with young children exposed to violence and other trauma* (2nd ed.). Zero to Three.

Lucio, R., & Nelson, T. L. (2016). Effective practices in the treatment of trauma in children and adolescents: From guidelines to organizational practices. *Journal of Evidence-Informed Social Work*, *13*(5), 469–478. https://doi.org/10.1080/23761407.2016.1166839

Lyons-Ruth, K., & Jacobvitz, D. (2016). Attachment disorganization from infancy to adulthood: Neurobiological correlates, parenting contexts, and pathways to disorder. In J. Cassidy & P. R. Shaver (Eds.), *Handbook of attachment: Theory, research, and clinical applications* (3rd ed., pp. 667–695). The Guilford Press.

Martin, A., Naunton, M., Kosari, S., Peterson, G., Thomas, J., & Christenson, J. K. (2021). Treatment guidelines for PTSD: A systematic review. *Journal of Clinical Medicine*, *10*(18), 4175. https://doi.org/10.3390/jcm10184175

Masud, H., Ahmad, M. S., Cho, K. W., & Fakhr, Z. (2019). Parenting styles and aggression among young adolescents: A systematic review of literature. *Community Mental Health Journal, 55*(6), 1015–1030. https://doi.org/10.1007/s10597-019-00400-0

Mavranezouli, I., Megnin-Viggars, O., Daly, C., Dias, S., Stockton, S., Meiser-Stedman, R., Trickey, D., & Pilling, S. (2020). Research Review: Psychological and psychosocial treatments for children and young people with post-traumatic stress disorder: A network meta-analysis. *Journal of Child Psychology and Psychiatry, and Allied Disciplines, 61*(1), 18–29. https://doi.org/10.1111/jcpp.13094

McLaughlin, K. A., & Lambert, H. K. (2018). Child trauma exposure and psychopathology: Mechanisms of risk and resilience. *Current Opinion in Psychology, 14*, 29–34. https://www.ncbi.nlm.nih.gov/pmc/articles/PMC5111863/

Messer, E. P., Greiner, M., Beal, S., Cassedy, A., Eismann, E., Gurwitch, R. H., Boat, B., Bensman, H., Bemerer, J., Greenwell, S., & Eiler-Sims, P. (2018). Child adult relationship enhancement (CARE): A brief, skills-building training for foster caregivers to increase positive parenting practices. *Children and Youth Services Review, 90*, 74–82. https://doi.org/10.1016/j.childyouth.2018.05.017

Mittelmark, M. B., & Bauer, G. F. (2022). Salutogenesis as a theory, as an orientation and as the sense of coherence. In M. B. Mittelmark, S. Sagy, M. Eriksson, G. Bauer, J. M. Pelikan, B. Lindström, & G. A. Espnes (Eds.), *The handbook of salutogenesis* (pp. 11–18). Springer Open.

National Institute for Care and Excellence (NICE). (2018). *Psychological interventions for prevention and treatment of children and young people.* https://www.nice.org.uk/guidance/ng116/chapter/Recommendations#management-of-ptsd-in-children-young-people-and-adults

O'Byrne, E., McCusker, C., & McSweeney, S. (2023). The impact of the "Attachment and Biobehavioural Catch-Up" program on attachment related parent behavior—A systematic review. *Infant Mental Health Journal, 44*, 76–91. https://doi.org/10.1002/imhj.22025

Olff, M., Monson, C. M., Riggs, D. S., Lee, C., Ehlers, A., & Forbes, D. (2020). Psychological treatments: Core and common elements of effectiveness. In D. Forbes, J. I. Bisson, C. M. Monson, & L. Berliner (Eds.), *Effective treatments for PTSD: Practice guidelines from the International Society for Traumatic Stress Studies* (pp. 169–187). The Guilford Press.

Osofsky, J. D., & Osofsky, H. J. (2018). Challenges in building child and family resilience after disasters. *Family Social Work, 21*, 115–128. https://doi.org/10.1080/10522158.2018.1427644

Powers, M. B., Halpern, J. M., Ferenschak, M. P., Gillihan, S. J., & Foa, E. B. (2010). A meta-analytic review of prolonged exposure for posttraumatic stress disorder. *Clinical Psychology Review, 30*(6), 635–641. https://doi.org/10.1016/j.cpr.2010.04.007

Rasines-Laudes, P., & Serrano-Pintado, I. (2023). Efficacy of EMDR in post-traumatic stress disorder: A systematic review and meta-analysis of randomized clinical trials. *Psicothema, 35*(4), 385–396. https://doi.org/10.7334/psicothema2022.309

Reddemann, L., & Piedfort-Marin, O. (2017). Stabilization in the treatment of complex post-traumatic stress disorders: Concepts and principles. *European Journal of Trauma & Dissociation, 1*(1), 11–17. https://doi.org/10.1016/j.ejtd.2017.01.009

Resick, P. A., Williams, L. F., Suvak, M. K., Monson, C. M., & Gradus, J. L. (2012). Long-term outcomes of cognitive-behavioral treatments for posttraumatic stress disorder among female rape survivors. *Journal of Consulting and Clinical Psychology, 80*(2), 201–210. https://doi.org/10.1037/a0026602

Roben, C. K. P., Dozier, M., Caron, E., & Bernard, K. (2017). Moving an evidence-based parenting program into the community. *Child Development, 88*, 1447–1452. https://doi.org/10.1111/cdev.12898

Sackett, D., Rosenberg, W., Gray, J., Haynes, R., & Richardson, W. (1996). Evidence-based medicine: What it is and what it isn't. *British Medical Journal, 312*(7023), 71–72. https://doi.org/10.1136/bmj.312.7023.71

Schilling, S., French, B., Berkowitz, S. J., Dougherty, S. L., Scribano, P. V., & Wood, J. N. (2016). Child-adult relationship enhancement in primary care (PriCARE): A randomized trial of a parent training for child behavior problems. *Academic Pediatrics, 17*(1), 53–60. https://doi.org/10.1016/j.acap.2016.06.009

Schnurr, P. P., Chard, K. M., Ruzek, J. I., Chow, B. K., Resick, P. A., Foa, E. B., Marx, B. P., Friedman, M. J., Bovin, M. J., Caudle, K. L., Castillo, D., Curry, K. T., Hollifield, M., Huang, G. D., Chee, C. L., Astin, M. C., Dickstein, B., Renner, K., Clancy, C. P., Collie, C., Maieritsch, K., Bailey, S., Thompson, K., Messina, M., Franklin, L., Lindley, S., Katter, K., Luedtke, B., Romesser, J., McQuaid, J., Sylvers, P., Varkovitzky, R., Davis, L., MacVicar, D., & Shih, M. C. (2022). Comparison of prolonged exposure vs cognitive processing therapy for treatment of posttraumatic stress disorder among US veterans: A randomized clinical trial. *JAMA Network Open, 5*(1), e2136921. https://doi.org/10.1001/jamanetworkopen.2021.36921

Schubert, S. J., Lee, C. W., & Drummond, P. D. (2010). The efficacy and psychophysiological correlates of dual-attention tasks in eye movement desensitization and reprocessing (EMDR). *Journal of Anxiety Disorders, 25*, 1–11. https://doi.org/10.1016/j.janxdis.2010.06.024

Sloan, D. M., Feinstein, B., Gallagher, M. W., Beck, J. G., & Keane, T. M. (2013). Efficacy of group treatment for posttraumatic stress disorder: A meta-analysis. *Psychological Trauma: Theory, Research, Practice, and Policy, 5*(2), 176–183. https://doi.org/10.1080/10503307.2017.1405168

Steele, K., Boon, S., & van der Hart, O. (2017). *Treating trauma-related dissociation: A practical, integrative approach.* W. W. Norton.

Tabachnick, A. R., Raby, K. L., Goldstein, A., Zajac, L., & Dozier, M. (2019). Effects of an attachment-based intervention in infancy on children's autonomic regulation during middle childhood. *Biological Psychology, 143*, 22. https://doi.org/10.1016/j.biopsycho.2019.01.006

The International Society of Traumatic Stress Studies (ISTSS). (2019). *ISTSS guidelines position paper on Complex PTSD in children and adolescents.* www.istss.org/getattachemen/Treating-Trauma/New-ISTSS-Prevention-and-Treatment-Guidelines/ISTSS_CPTSD-Position-Paper-(Children-and-Adolescents)_FNL.pdf.aspx

Thomas, F. C., Loskot, T., Mutschler, C., Burdo, J., Lagdamen, J., Sijercic, I., Lane, J. E. M., Liebman, R. E., Finley, E. P., Monson, C. M., & Wiltsey-Stirman, S. (2023). Initiative Cognitive-Processing Therapy (CPT) in community settings: A qualitative investigation of therapist decision-making. *Administration and Policy in Mental Health, 50,* 137–150. https://doi.org/10.1007/s10488-022-01229-8

VA/DoD Clinical Practice Guideline Working Group. (2017). *VA/DoD clinical practice guideline for the management of posttraumatic stress disorder and acute stress disorder.* VA Office of Quality and Performance.

VA/DoD Clinical Practice Guideline Working Group. (2023). *VA/DoD clinical practice guideline for the management of posttraumatic stress disorder and acute stress disorder.* VA Office of Quality and Performance.

Valadez, E. A., Tottenham, N., Tabachnick, A. R., & Dozier, M. (2020). Early parenting intervention effects on brain responses to maternal cues among high-risk children. *American Journal of Psychiatry, 177*(9), 818–826. https://doi.org/10.1176/appi.ajp.2020.20010011

van den Hout, M. A., Engelhard, I. M., Beetsma, D., Slofstra, C., Hornsveld, H., Houtveen, J., & Leer, A. (2011). EMDR and mindfulness: Eye movements and attentional breathing tax working memory and reduce vividness and emotionality of aversive ideation. *Journal of Behavior Therapy and Experimental Psychiatry, 42,* 423e431. https://doi.org/10.1016/j.jbtep.2011.03.004

van der Velden, P. G., Grievink, L., Kleber, R. J., Drogendijk, A. N., Roskam, A. J., Marcelissen, F. G., Olff, M., Meewisse, M. L., & Gersons, B. P. (2006). Post-disaster mental health problems and the utilization of mental health services: A four-year longitudinal comparative study. *Administration and Policy in Mental Health, 33*(3), 279–288. https://doi.org/10.1007/s10488-005-0027-x

Wampold, B. E. (2015). How important are the common factors in psychotherapy? An update. *World Psychiatry, 14*(3), 270–277. https://doi.org/10.1002/wps.20238

Watkins, L. E., Sprang, K. R., & Rothbaum, B. O. (2018). Treating PTSD: A review of evidence-based psychotherapy interventions. *Frontiers in Behavioral Neuroscience, 12,* 258. https://doi.org/10.3389/fnbeh.2018.00258

References

Chapter Seven
Suicide, Crisis, and Disaster

Overview

Suicide, attempts, and non-suicidal self-injury are significant concerns for helpers, but the need for emergency responders during crises or disasters is great. Chapter 7: Suicide, Crisis, and Disaster focuses on the unpredictability, safety, and resilience in the face of crisis. This chapter discusses suicide assessment, non-suicidal self-injury, and ways to help those with suicidal ideation. The discussion spoke of suicide risk factors and the need for developing a trauma-informed suicide assessment. Chapter 7 continues with models of crisis and disaster responses, including a brief explanation of the 7-Stage Crisis Intervention model, Psychological First Aid, and Critical Incident Stress Management/Critical Incident Stress Debriefing. The chapter ends with a focus on resilience and adaptive responses to crises and disasters.

When Crisis Strikes

Many people desire a peaceful and worry-free life. Others enjoy being spontaneous, being surprised by something wonderful, such as the birth of a new child, or receiving an unexpected gift. The feeling of safety comes when life is predictable. However, moments arrive when circumstances bring chaos and devastation. These challenge our determination and flexibility. We may view these as uncomfortable but as opportunities for growth. When a crisis or disaster arrives, the added stressors or burdens that require increased energy and resolve may consume us. Our perseverance through difficult times is contingent, in part, on our perception and interpretation of these events. It also depends on resource availability. If our view of the catastrophe is dismal and

DOI: 10.4324/9781003463009-7

we lack the resources to manage it, the negative impact will intensify. One only needs to look back to 2019, when COVID-19 arrived, to witness such a cataclysmic situation.

With little knowledge of the coronavirus, how to manage it, and a lack of resources, many felt betrayed by the systems designed to offer protection and guidance. This collective trauma descended as a dark cloud and changed the way we think and do things. The consequences of COVID-19 not only caused death and long-term physical effects but also created psychological distress. Frontline healthcare professionals and mental health providers were unprepared for the upheaval (Mehedi & Ismail Hossain, 2022; Slone et al., 2021). Suicide rates increased during the COVID-19 pandemic, as well as mental health problems (Negri et al., 2023; Pathirathna et al., 2022). This natural disaster reminded all of us that life may be unpredictable. Crises affect everyone; not just those faced with a personal crisis, but also those who care and support that person. As helpers, we must expect, prepare for, and manage these situations as they occur through a trauma-sensitive lens. These unlikely situations are far more common than we expect, and people deal with suicidal thoughts or gestures, crises, or disasters daily.

Suicide Prevention and Intervention

Denise recalls her training in suicide prevention and intervention. In graduate school, other students recommended training with a local suicide prevention agency. She registered for the seminar, which included 20–25 hours of psychoeducation about suicide and 40 hours of role play. Upon completion, Denise signed up for overnight shifts every Friday with a friend. She remembers how nervous she was to work that first time. What if she made a mistake? It did not take long for her to make that first gaffe. The night was quiet, and Denise drifted to sleep. She heard the ring ring of the phone and answered it. However, she was not quite awake, so her immediate response was from a part-time job. "Hello, First State Mortgage. How can I help you?" As Denise uttered the words aloud, she realized that was not the correct answer. The person calling said, "I was trying to reach the suicide hotline." Flustered, Denise replied, "Oh, I am so sorry. This *is* it. I apologize. Yes, you have called Suicide Prevention. How can I help you?" Denise never made *that* mistake again. However, she made other errors. Nonetheless, Denise was faithful to that shift and helped save lives.

When a helper faces a person with suicidal ideation, it can be unnerving. Some of the most anxious moments for helpers are those involving clients who are suicidal. Whether you are a licensed therapist, police officer, nurse, educator, or emergency worker, you will assist someone who is thinking of harming themselves. Assessing people who are a suicide risk elicits powerful emotions. That probably means you will experience anxiety, tension, or fear. You may have negative feelings or thoughts about those who are suicidal. Some trauma workers feel helpless, hopeless, troubled, or worried (Bühlmann et al., 2021). Nevertheless, your actions may save a life. This makes suicidal awareness, intervention, and prevention a critical area of focus.

Frequency, Risk Factors, and Warning Signs

Suicide is a global issue, and when providers miss intervention, it results in a 30% fatality rate (Barzilay et al., 2018). Suicide rates increased between 1999 and 2017 from 10.5 per 100,000 to 14.0 per 100,000 people, representing a 33% rise (Hedegaard et al., 2018). In the United States, suicide is within the top 10 leading causes of death (American Foundation for Suicide Prevention, 2019). In 2017 and 2020, suicide was the second-highest cause of death among adolescents and young adults (Curtin & Heron, 2019; Hughes et al., 2023). The methods most used are firearms, which comprise almost 44% of all deaths among 10–19-year-olds, and hanging or suffocation, accounting for 43% of all deaths (Hughes et al., 2023).

Risk factors for suicide are multifaceted and related to individual health and environmental factors. Other risk factors include a history of psychiatric diagnoses, prior suicide attempts, a family history of suicide, recent stressors, access to lethal means, and non-suicidal self-harm (Castellví et al., 2017; Chen et al., 2024; Keyes et al., 2024). Social demographics, such as age, gender, race, and poverty level, relate to suicidality. Adolescents and older adults are at an increased risk (Glenn et al., 2020). Risk factors for medical students who have high suicide rates include heavy academic stress or pressure, academic failure, harassment, hazing, or bullying, a prior psychiatric condition, past suicide attempts, and relational problems (Varshney et al., 2024). Rates of suicide among male youth are three times higher than among females, but suicidal ideation, suicidal planning, and non-fatal suicide attempts are higher in females (Keyes et al., 2024; Xiao et al., 2023). Suicide rates are higher for American Indians/Alaskan Natives and sexual minorities, people who identify as having same-sex attraction, being transgender, or gender-fluid (Hughes et al., 2023).

One pressing concern is predicting suicide. How can providers know when an individual may be at the most significant risk? Unfortunately, for the past 50 years, mental health providers and researchers have not been successful at predicting suicidal behaviors or suicide attempts (Franklin et al., 2017). Most suicide planning occurs within 12 hours of an attempt (Millner et al., 2020). Warning signs, or detectable cues that a person is at an increased risk, include talking about or making plans, expressing hopelessness, experiencing unbearable emotional distress, and marked changes in behavior. Other warning signs of youth are withdrawal, sleep problems, and risky behavior (King et al., 2023). Rudd et al. (2006) identify ten warning signs for heightened risk: suicide ideation, substance abuse, purposelessness, anger, feeling trapped, hopelessness, withdrawal, anxiety, recklessness, and mood change. However, there is little evidence that these are true of all suicidal people. For psychiatric adult inpatients, risk factors include lifetime suicide attempts and recency of attempts. The most identified factor is hopelessness, followed by anxiety and intense emotional pain (Tsai & Klonsky, 2023). Recent studies show that the number of behavioral warning signs indicates an increased risk for suicide attempts (Littlefield et al., 2024).

To determine risk, several models have helped identify common factors and pathways to a suicide attempt. One such model is the interpersonal theory of suicide, which poses that suicidal ideation occurs when a person perceives they are unable to manage life, experience intrapsychic pain, and have lost connection with others. According to this theory, suicidal ideation arises when a person perceives an inability to manage life, experiences emotional pain, and loses connection with others (Klonsky et al., 2017; Van Orden et al., 2008). The three-step theory of suicide explains the process of suicide while differentiating between suicidal ideators and suicidal attempters. This ideation-to-action framework states that suicidal ideation occurs from a combination of pain and hopelessness. Activation of suicidal thoughts occurs with an imbalance of pain versus connection and progresses from suicidal thoughts to actions, which are moderated by disposition, learned behaviors, and practical factors (Klonsky et al., 2017). Another model is the integrated motivational-volitional (IMV) model, which states that a sense of defeat and entrapment are key mediators (O'Connor & Portzky, 2018). According to the IMV model, helpers need to assess suicidal ideation, intent, and behaviors, including past suicidal behavior, mental imagery, fearlessness of death, physical pain sensitivity or endurance, impulsivity, exposure to suicide or suicidal behavior, suicidal plan formulation, and access to lethal means. While suicide prediction scales exist, they offer little reassurance to helpers due to the poor accuracy in suicide prediction (Zortea et al., 2020). This means that suicide assessment must incorporate the use of suicide assessment tools and a psychosocial assessment.

When Crisis Strikes

Suicide Assessment and Intervention

Practical suicide assessment explores the complete history of health, life stressors, relationships, and coping strategies through a clinical interview, which reduces the risk of self-harm, and a suicide screening instrument (Zortea et al., 2020). The screening alone is unreliable in preventing suicide but helps determine contributing factors, plans, intent, and resources needed. It also allows the full opportunity to develop an individualized safety plan with the suicidal person. Since suicide is multifactorial, the interventions must be multifaceted as well (Chen et al., 2024).

While working in a psychiatric hospital, John discovered he knew less about suicide than he realized. Previously, he worked as an outpatient mental health therapist in a private practice. Whenever John had a patient who was suicidal, he would send the patient to the psychiatric hospital for admission, expecting them to stay. Then John would be angry when they showed up at his office or called him the following day, stating they were not admitted. "Why didn't they keep you?" The client explained that the hospital had said they did not need to be there. John often blamed the hospital staff, stating they must be incompetent. However, when he began working in admissions at the psychiatric hospital, he got a first-hand look at what was happening. Clients like his former ones would walk in for an assessment, being referred by their therapists, and they would assess them for suicide. However, once they were at the hospital, these clients would decide they did not want to be there and would answer the questions in such a way that the hospital could not keep them. They might admit they thought about suicide earlier in the day or a few days ago, but not now. They would be vague about any plan and would deny they had access to lethal weapons or pills and had no intent. They would deny previous attempts or hospitalizations. Under those conditions, the hospital could not keep them. If only the therapist had signed a third-party statement and sent it beforehand. John was frustrated with the therapist. His hands were tied, and John knew that once the client returned, the therapist would be angry and think he was incompetent. There was no way to win. Worst of all, he was concerned that the client was a danger to themself. Indeed, there was a better way to do this. This is why coordination of care is so important for ensuring patient safety.

While multiple assessments and interventions exist, few incorporate a trauma-informed perspective. However, people who attempt suicide have elevated rates of trauma exposure. When helpers are unaware of the trauma exposure, their responses may be harmful, cause the suicidal person to feel unsafe, and prevent the interventions from being useful (Asarnow et al., 2020). To address this problem, Adams et al. (2022) developed an approach that integrates the core components of trauma-informed care and the 7-Stage Crisis Intervention Model (SSCIM). The SSCIM is a crisis intervention model that includes assessment, collaborative relationships, identification of problems and precipitants, emotional exploration, generativity of alternatives and coping strategies, implementation of an action plan, and follow-up (Roberts & Ottens, 2005). While ensuring safety, the helper must also know how their decisions about client safety affect the client's autonomy, how those decisions might re-traumatize the client, and how it will impact their relationship with the client (Akther et al., 2020). Inpatient hospitalization, emergency departments, and medical transportation for suicidal people are destabilizing and may cause re-traumatization (Saunders et al., 2023). If possible, completing a thorough assessment and stabilizing the person is the preferred course of action.

Another model intervention, while not trauma-informed but valuable, is the Crisis Response Plan (Bryan et al., 2017). The Crisis Response Plan uses a multifaceted intervention with evidence that shows a 76% reduction in suicidal behavior. It helps reduce emotional distress and inpatient psychiatric days, increases optimism, and can be easily adapted to psychotherapeutic care (Rozek & Bryan, 2020). When completing safety planning, identify individual warning signs, coping skills, reasons for living, support networks, resources, and professional crisis referrals (Rozek & Bryan, 2020). While no-suicide contracts have been used in the past, there is little evidence that they protect the suicidal person. Instead, they may be harmful, causing further risk for suicidal behaviors and increasing one's liability (Edwards & Sachmann, 2010) (Figure 7.1).

Assessment tools for screening are readily available. The Columbia Suicide Severity Rating Scale (C-SSRS) is the most highly recommended tool to measure current and past suicidal ideation, attempts, preparatory behaviors, and non-suicidal self-injury. The instrument comes in assessment form, including a psychosocial assessment and a quick screen. Research by Horwitz et al. (2014) suggests that a more extended assessment is associated with better outcomes in prediction. Another model is the Assess, Intervene, and Monitor for Suicide Prevention (AIM-SP), which offers screening, comprehensive risk assessment, brief psychosocial interventions, and strategies for ongoing monitoring (Brodsky et al., 2018).

When Crisis Strikes

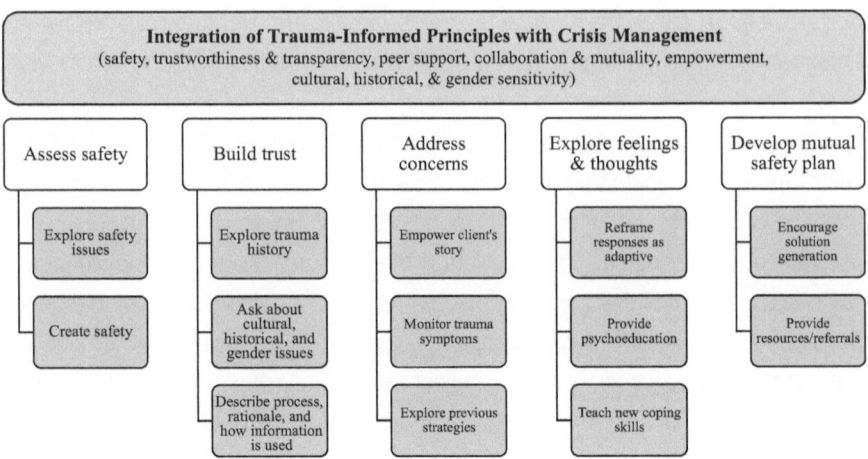

FIGURE 7.1 Integration of Trauma-Informed Principles with Crisis Management. (Adapted from Bryan et al., 2017; Rozek & Bryan, 2020).

Assessing Self-Harm

Determining safety should include an assessment of non-suicidal self-injury (NSSI), which is the deliberate, self-inflicted harm to one's body that is not culturally or socially accepted (Carr et al., 2017; Westers & Plener, 2020). This is vital because of the high risk of suicide related to self-harm. In adolescents and young adults, NSSI accounts for 26% of future suicide attempts. Studies determined that there is a 70–80-fold increase in the risk of future suicide attempts for those people who self-harm (Castellví et al., 2017). In the United States, there is an increasing lifetime prevalence of NSSI in adolescents, especially those aged 10–14 years (Bell et al., 2016). To date, no tool accurately assesses self-harm or serves as an appropriate intervention. People often stigmatize and view individuals who self-harm as attention seekers, needy, and undeserving of additional time. Often, patients with NSSI are shamed, punished, or refused care when they need the most support (Mughal et al., 2023). This is a problem because the lack of proper assessment can lead to further self-harm and suicide (Quinlivan et al., 2022). The National Institute for Health and Care Excellence (NICE) guides the assessment and intervention of NSSI. They recommend against using a risk assessment but emphasize the need for a comprehensive psychosocial assessment. This is due to the poor instruments available to assess self-harm, which may misinform providers that a person is safe when they are not (Chaplin, 2023; NICE, 2022). Instead, helpers need to focus on providing a compassionate, non-judgmental, and empathic approach that seeks to determine the method of self-harm, the frequency and cause of self-harm, and a collaborative plan of safety. The assessment should foster hope for the person and determine the resources needed to maintain safety (Mughal et al., 2023).

Nurture Understanding

Tyler had been to the hospital several times. He hated to go, but his family insisted. Tyler tried to hide the cuts and burns, but his sister usually found him. This time he cut so deep he could not stop the bleeding on his stomach. As Tyler walked in the emergency department, he saw the clerk roll her eyes and then turn to her co-worker and mouth the words, "It's him again." Tyler felt such shame. He knew they hated him. Tyler checked in and then waited for two hours even though there were few people in the emergency room. When the doctor walked in to check him, he didn't even look at Tyler. The doctor didn't ask what happened. He checked the wound, dressed it, and said, "You need to stop this." And then the doctor just walked out. Tyler started crying. His sister patted him on the back, but she also said, "Tyler, I just don't understand you." Tyler wanted to tell them all, "Don't you think I want to stop? Don't you know that what you say just makes me want to kill myself?" However, he did not say anything. Tyler does not dare to kill himself – yet. Maybe someday he will. Today, Tyler wants to go home and be by himself. He feels so alone.

- As you read Tyler's story, what thoughts come to you?
- In what way is stigmatization preventing Tyler from receiving the care he needs?
- What judgment words or phrases have you heard about suicidal clients?

Other clients have similar stories to Tyler. How sad that these clients are treated with such disdain. Yet, this is quite common. In emergency departments, lengthy waiting times with little communication, lack of individualized care, superficial contact with little sensitivity, stigmatization, mistrust, and lack of compassion toward patients who self-harm are expected (Uddin et al., 2023).

Suicide Prevention Strategies

Prevention strategies for suicide lack research to support their efficacy. In suicide prevention programs, knowledge and intervention strategies are the most researched aspects. Improvement rates in knowledge and self-efficacy are notable.

When Crisis Strikes

While these may reduce suicide, the problem remains with coordination of care (Barnhorst et al., 2021). Protective factors for suicide include problem-focused coping skills, task-oriented coping strategies, and positive self-worth. Healthy lifestyles are related to less suicidal ideation in adults, but not adolescents. A secure attachment with family or friends may be protective, but studies show mixed results, with higher protection for suicidal females only (Bakken et al., 2024). A third approach is the Suicide Assessment Five-step Evaluation and Triage (SAFE-T), which identifies risk and protective factors, suicidal thoughts, plans, behaviors, intentions, risk levels, and interventions (Rico, 2016). For adolescents, the SAFETY-A steps include adopting a trauma-informed stance, protecting and establishing physical and psychological safety, recognizing trauma exposure, mobilizing peer, family, and community resources, conducting a trauma-informed assessment, using trauma interventions, and monitoring for adverse effects. The plan invites families to participate in identifying the suicidal youth's strengths, emotional reactions, engagement in safety planning, safe people, and commitment to following the safety plan (Asarnow et al., 2020).

Cultivate Knowledge

Janet calls you on Friday at 4:45 p.m. You are ready to go home and have plans for the evening. However, Janet tells you she is not sure she wants to be here anymore. She does not think anyone cares about her. This is not new for Janet. She often struggles with these thoughts. She has been hospitalized in the past from a suicide attempt and frequently cuts herself:

- How do you proceed with this call?
- What questions would you ask Janet?
- What action steps would you take?

In assessment, treatment, and prevention efforts, a trauma-sensitive approach will incorporate the principles of trauma-informed care. This means acknowledging that the person in need may have trauma exposure, traumatic stress symptoms, or PTSD. Despite the stress, care providers should monitor their physiological arousal and regulate their emotional state when helping. In doing so, they can offer physical and emotional safety, build trust, provide transparency, and develop a collaborative and mutual bond with the person needing aid. A trauma-informed approach to suicidal ideation, attempts, and NSSI means empowering patients to determine the best route to health and acknowledging how their social network, culture, gender, and history contribute to wellness. While suicide, suicidal behaviors, and non-suicidal self-injury constitute a significant concern for helpers, the need for emergency responders during crises or disasters is great.

Stages of Crises and Disasters

Everyone faces a crisis at one point or another. Disasters, whether natural or human-initiated, will occur. The nature of crises and disasters means that they happen without warning, are uncontrollable, and cause people to feel vulnerable. A typical cycle ensues with disorganization and disequilibrium, wherein people are frustrated with delays in responses and the ambiguity of the situation. There is shock, fear, and distress. Such events challenge everyone's coping skills. What some view as a crisis, others will see as just everyday events. This means a crisis is related to individual perceptions and experiences of an arduous situation. However, when one person experiences a crisis, it affects those around them. Usually, crises are time-limited, but the effects of such can last a lifetime.

The three primary frameworks for crisis intervention are the equilibrium, cognitive, and psychosocial transition models. According to the equilibrium model, when a crisis arrives, people experience a psychological state of flux or emotional disequilibrium with insufficient resources. The primary focus of this model is stabilization (Caplan, 1964). Presupposing that how one perceives crises depends on pre-existing schemes, not on the event, facts, or situation, is the cognitive model of crisis intervention. This model aims to increase individual awareness of the need for change in faulty thinking (Meichenbaum, 1995). The psychosocial transition model, by contrast, proposes that genetics and learning influence how people respond to crises. This outlook considers the individual, family, and systemic influences that either contribute to or hinder growth. Whichever model one applies in crisis or disaster counseling, the need is for immediacy, stabilization, symptom reduction, and a return to adaptive functioning (Ahmad, 2019).

Interventions During Crises or Disasters

Situations arise that are crises or disasters. Crisis and trauma are different. Caplan (1961) states that a crisis is a temporary obstacle that seems unbeatable using typical problem-solving skills. A period of disequilibrium accompanies it, which results in disorganization and distress. While a crisis may lead to traumatic symptoms, most people can restore their functioning to pre-crisis when they have the right resources (Adams et al., 2022). A disaster, which natural events or human-initiated actions can cause, occurs suddenly, and disrupts a population, resulting in loss of life, resources, and economy (James & Gilliland, 2016). Offering help during crises or following disasters differs from providing counseling or therapy. Crisis work is time-limited, and a helper must build rapport rapidly with the goal of moving the client from immobility to mobility and return to a pre-crisis state. There is no in-depth exploration of issues during a crisis (Pau et al., 2020).

These critical incidents occur in a person's or community's life without warning and can be emotionally challenging. Whether a crisis or disaster leads to PTSD may depend on the help offered. Early support may decrease the symptoms or the duration of symptoms but requires that teams receive preparation and training prior to such events. Critical incidents are common and cause powerful physical and psychological reactions in individuals and groups. These incidents may include events that involve serious illness, injury, or death of children, co-workers, or family members. They may be work-related injuries, deaths, suicides, or shootings. Others may be threats of violence, accidents, medical errors that injure patients, damage people or equipment, or hazardous materials that jeopardize lives or equipment. A crisis causes an acute emotional reaction due to a potent stimulus (Mitchell & Everly, 2023). Humans or natural forces can cause disasters. Natural disasters, such as tornados, hurricanes, floods, and others, can be devastating, causing a loss of lives, homes, possessions, communities, and the economy. Disasters caused by humans may include terrorism or war, or technological or accidental in nature and can result in multiple losses (Kusmaul, 2021). Whether the losses are because of a crisis or disaster, the needs are the same: safety, calm, self and community efficacy, connection, and hope (Hobfoll et al., 2007). As a helper, you can provide these for those in crisis and your co-workers with some pre-training.

Emergency Interventions

Responding to those who experience crises or disasters may take much work. Instead, the situation may require a holistic view that encompasses understanding the community's needs, the potential problems, what facilitates community healing, and factors that diminish future vulnerability (Rosenberg et al., 2022). In working with individuals and communities who experience crises or disasters, the Substance Abuse and Mental Health Services Administration (SAMHSA) recommends that all responders keep four trauma-informed principles in mind:

- Realize that trauma affects people and groups.
- Recognize how trauma may show up in interpersonal interactions and relationships.
- Respond with supportive, caring, and trauma-informed care and communication.
- Avoid re-traumatization by responding to survivors and team members in compassionate and supportive ways.

(SAMHSA, 2014)

To do so, several training programs are offered to ensure these elements are in place when offering services during emergent situations.

Psychological First Aid

Introduced shortly after World War II, Psychological First Aid (PFA) was developed as an initial form of support for those people who experienced a severe stressor. It was designed to provide information, comfort, practical assistance, and referral to additional services if needed (Hermosilla et al., 2023; Wang et al., 2021). The principles of PFA follow Hobfoll's five principles for mass trauma interventions (Hobfoll et al., 2007) based on Maslow's hierarchy of needs, addressing physical and safety needs first before attending to psychological needs (Maslow, 1943). The PFA is not a form of therapy but is intended to provide practical assistance and stabilization. There are six steps, with the first three focused on attending, observing, and understanding the individual's problem. The last three steps are action-oriented and designed to engage the client in taking steps to regain control and autonomy (James & Gilliland, 2016). There are several types of PFA, but the three most common are WHO-PFA, NCTSN-PFA, and Johns Hopkins RAPID-PFA, all of which are manual versions. While there is little evidence of the positive effect of PFA, this does not mean it is an ineffective protocol. It does provide workers with knowledge and skills to ensure a universal approach to a crisis. Studies showed that it increases the confidence of helpers in providing aid (Wang et al., 2021).

Stages of Crises and Disasters

Immediate Post-Crisis Interventions

The three most used post-trauma interventions are Critical Incident Stress Debriefing (CISD; Mitchell, 1983), psychological debriefing (Dyregov & Regel, 2012), and trauma risk management (TRiM; Jones et al., 2017). In 2005, the National Institute for Clinical Excellence (NICE) determined there was insufficient evidence that these decreased PTSD symptoms. However, it acknowledged that psychological debriefing was an excellent practice following a traumatic incident. However, NICE updated this guideline in 2018, stating that brief, single-session interventions were not recommended (National Guideline Alliance, 2018; Richins et al., 2020). Watson and Andrews (2018) stated that TRiM was more effective in aiding recovery than general debriefing and other early interventions. However, success rates depend on the support of the managers and supervisors and reduced stigma placed on receiving the protocol (Jones et al., 2017; Watson & Andrews, 2018).

Critical Incident Stress Management and Debriefing

Mitchell created Critical Incident Stress Management and Debriefing to address the needs created by crises. The goals of CISM/CISD are to stabilize the situation, reduce emotional tension and distress, mobilize resources, lessen the event impact, normalize reactions, restore adaptive function, facilitate the recovery process, restore unit cohesion and performance, and identify the need for additional care. Seven principles of crisis intervention exist: simplicity, brevity, innovation, pragmatism, proximity, immediacy, and expectancy (Mitchell & Everly, 2023).

A chaplain described his experience with CISM/CISD:

> I heard the gunshot outside my window. I work in a hospital, so I knew what happened. I was afraid to look outside but knew I needed to go out. Instead of looking, I ran outside to the front, where a crowd had gathered. I made my way through the crowd and found the veteran crumpled on the ground. The scene was terrible. I led the people away from the horrific scene while the first responders came to gather the body and clean the mess. I knew the veteran. He had been by my office several times. Life was much too complicated. Many had tried to help him. The guilt was heavy on all of us. I met with the administration later, and we made plans for the CISDs. My staff was trained and ready. Over the next 48 hours, we had several debriefings. They were hard, but the staff was appreciative. That was not the end.

Throughout the next few weeks, the staff stopped by my office or would stop the chaplains asking to talk. They shared their experience, or just about their lives, just wanting to connect on a human level, realizing that life was just too short. Some needed guidance, others recompense. We offered hope, forgiveness, and a kind word. We had a bond of woundedness and healing.

This powerful story demonstrates how offering a moment of CISD and the follow-up period can heal a traumatic experience.

CISD is one of the earliest interventions for psychological debriefing used to decrease immediate distress following a traumatic incident. It uses a semi-structured group setting with a trained group leader and peer support representative. It typically lasts approximately 1–3 hours and occurs 24–72 hours after the critical incident (Scott et al., 2022). There has been concern that CISD could cause harm, mainly due to a one-session debriefing with no follow-up sessions (National Guideline Alliance (UK), 2018). When CISD offers an acknowledgment of the psychological impact of trauma exposure, reassurance, validation of normal distress, and referral resources, along with an appropriate follow-up, then it becomes a helpful form of post-crisis intervention. It can then possibly reduce PTSD symptom severity and stress-related absences from work (Richins et al., 2020; Scott et al., 2022).

Tending Your Technique

When we teach, we often assign students to complete crisis intervention training for further skill development. Several online programs offer suicide training or crisis intervention training. Find one to complete and then respond to the following:

- What training did you complete?
- Describe three facts you learned that were new to you.
- List three actions you would consider using during a crisis or disaster.

A Flourishing Focus

No one wishes harm would come upon an individual or a community. Fred recalled being present when Mount St. Helens erupted in May 1980. At the time Fred worked in a hospital setting 150 miles from the epicenter and he remembers the subsequent eruptions, which resulted in ashes covering his car in the parking lot. Fred grieved about how this event had affected his community. Another businessman, Tom, recalled the tragedy of 9/11. His office was across the island from the World Trade Center, and he watched as the Towers collapsed. He lost business contacts and friends on that day. No matter where one lives, you will be near those who witness or survive catastrophic events. You may have survived tornados, earthquakes, and floods or have aided those who survived mass shootings and bombings. While heartbreaking, what most amazes us is how people rise above the loss and devastation. They rebuild their lives, their homes, and their communities.

Their resilience is astounding. Make no mistake. Resilience is not about bouncing back. That is a misunderstanding. Humans are not meant to return to the previous state, nor are their communities. They adapt, change, reorganize, and recreate (Walker, 2020). If a human or community remains the same, they have gained little from adversity. Resilience means learning how to change and resist future disturbances so that individuals, families, cultures, and systems can be stronger and maintain their integrity. It means recalibration through adaptive coping.

Unfortunately, when crises or disasters occur, the distress that individuals experience directly impacts others, spreading like a contagious disease and increasing anxiety even in those who are not directly affected. This is further aided by vast media coverage that provides provocative images, disaster narratives, dismal metrics, and forecasts of the negative consequences. While this occurs, few acknowledge the psychological resilience that arises during these times. This is called a resilience blind spot (Bonanno, 2021). For example, New York City health officials predicted a widespread mental health crisis after the 9/11 crisis, with the Federal Emergency Management Agency (FEMA) setting aside millions of dollars to aid those needing counseling. While many people did need help, it was not to the degree expected (Bonanno, 2021). The collective interactions of people and the relational support provided the security, identity, and cohesion needed (Calo-Blanco et al., 2017). As people worked together amid the disruption, they wove a story of resilience and strength (Quinn et al., 2021). People adjust in wonderfully unique ways during disasters. In her novel *My Sister's Keeper*, Jodi Picoult states, "The human capacity for burden is like bamboo – far more flexible than you would ever believe at first glance" (2004, p. 236). Bonanno et al. (2024) suggest that people are flexible in responding to dire situations through a flexible mindset and sequence. They state that this real-time process allows individuals to optimize strategies in response to current challenges (Bonanno et al., 2024).

While offering crisis and disaster care, we ought to attune to and broadcast stories of psychological resilience. In that way, we might bring hope to those who are struggling, and, despite the circumstances, these individuals can also use their adaptive capacities to re-order their world. This calibration occurs through posttraumatic growth when individuals or systems see new possibilities, find new ways of relating to one another, discover an appreciation of life, find personal strength, or deepen their spiritual forces. According to Altinsoy and Aypay (2021), individuals engage in problem-focused coping by employing action-oriented strategies to solve problems. They look for deeper meaning in adversity and through their affiliative bonds (Feldman, 2020). They awaken to a new life that is fresh and full of color. That is the power of resilience.

Gather Self-Awareness

As you have learned about suicide, crises, and disasters in this chapter, think about how this information affected your thinking, emotions, and physical sensations. Complete these sentences.

- When I think about working with someone who is suicidal, I become …
- If a crisis occurred at my workplace, I might …
- During the last disaster in my community, I experienced …

Chapter Summary

Chapter 7 explored the intricate and multifaceted nature of handling crises, disasters, suicide prevention, and intervention. It emphasized the impact of unexpected events on individuals and communities, highlighting the need for a trauma-informed approach to address the psychological distress that arises. The chapter discussed the increased suicide rates and mental health problems during the COVID-19 pandemic, emphasizing the importance of understanding risk factors, warning signs, and predictive models for suicide. It also stressed the significance of suicide assessment, intervention, and prevention strategies, urging the use of trauma-informed care and crisis intervention models to provide support effectively. While the 7-Stage Crisis Intervention Model is a beginning, there is still a further need for clinicians to research and quantify evidence-based models for suicide assessments that incorporate trauma-sensitive measures that incorporate a compassionate, non-judgmental approach.

Chapter 7 focused on the unpredictability, safety, and resilience in the face of crisis. It also described the differences between crises, natural disasters, and human-initiated disasters and their effects on individuals and communities. Several approaches were briefly explained, including Psychological First Aid and Critical Incident Stress Management/Critical Incident Stress Debriefing. Finally, this chapter explored the concept of resilience, the resilient blind spot, and how individuals and communities experience posttraumatic growth after crises and disasters. The chapter emphasized the adaptive capacity of individuals and communities to overcome adversity and find new ways of relating to one another, even in the face of crises and disasters. It also provided resources and references for further training and understanding in suicide prevention, crisis intervention, and disaster response.

Chapter Review

Please respond to the following questions.

- What are the risk factors for suicide, and how do they vary across different demographics?
- What are the common warning signs for heightened suicide risk?
- What is Psychological First Aid, and how does it differ from traditional therapy?
- How do individuals and communities demonstrate resilience after a crisis or disaster? What factors contribute to posttraumatic growth?

Key Term Assessment

Review the following terms and try to explain each concept.

- Suicide Assessment
- Non-suicide self-injury (NSSI)
- Crisis
- Disaster

- Psychological First Aid
- Critical Incident Stress Management/Critical Incident Stress Debriefing

Resources

The following resources may be helpful. At the time of this writing, they were accessible through the links provided.

- Alternatives to Suicide is a peer-based response that supports those who experience suicidal thoughts or have made attempts. It was developed by The Wildflower Alliance in the U.S. It offers online support groups, community forums, training, and research. https://alt2su-nsw.net
- General Services Administration. (2023). Trauma-informed disaster response course. https://www.performance.gov/cx/life-experiences/recovering-from-a-disaster/outputs/1/

  This site was co-created with federal response staff to provide interactive education with videos, worksheets, and a guidebook to strengthen disaster recovery response.
- Psychological First Aid (PFA). (2024). The National Child Trauma Services Network (NCTSN) provides this five-hour interactive course to learn the core goals of PFA. https://www.nctsn.org/resources/psychological-first-aid-pfa-online
- The Columbia Lighthouse Project offers information about and training in suicide prevention. It uses the Columbia Protocol. The site provides the Columbia-Suicide Severity Rating Scale (C-SSRS). https://cssrs.columbia.edu/about-the-project/about-the-lighthouse-project/
- The National Empowerment Center is a website dedicated to recovery, empowerment, hope, and healing for people living with mental health issues, trauma, or extreme states. It offers resources, articles, information, crisis alternatives, videos, and newsletters. https://power2u.org
- The Stanley-Brown Safety Planning Intervention is a brief and collaborative intervention between the helper and the person with suicidality. It offers training, forms, and resources. https://suicidesafetyplan.com
- Zero Suicide offers self-paced online courses to increase knowledge and skills in suicide prevention. The courses are free. The Education Development Center

developed them through partnerships with the Suicide Prevention Resource Center and the Substance Abuse and Mental Health Services Administration. https://zerosuicidetraining.edc.org

References

Adams, C. R., Blueford, J. M., & Diambra, J. F. (2022). Trauma-informed crisis intervention. *Journal of Professional Counseling: Practice, Theory & Research, 49*(2), 91–107. https://doi. org/10.1080/15566382.2022.2148810

Ahmad, N. S. (2019). Crisis intervention: Issues and challenges. *Advances in Social Science, Education and Humanities Research* (*ASSEHR*), 304, 452–455. Doi: 10.2991/ acpch-18.2019.105

Akther, S. F., Molyneaux, E., Stuart, R., Johnson, S., Simpson, A., & Oram, S. (2020). Patients experiences of assessment and detention under mental health legislation: Systematic review and qualitative meta-synthesis. *BJPsych Open, 5*(3), e37. https://doi.org/10.1192/bjo.2019.19

Altinsoy, F., & Aypay, A. (2021). A post-traumatic growth model: Psychological hardiness, happiness-increasing strategies, and problem-focused coping. *Current Psychology, 42,* 2208–2220. https://doi.org/10.1007/s12144-021-02466-0

American Foundation for Suicide Prevention. (2019). *Together saving lives 2019 annual report.* https://annual2019.afsp.org/pdfs/AFSP-AnnualReport-web.pdf

Asarnow, J. R., Goldston, D. B., Tunno, A. M., Inscoe, A. B., & Pynoos, R. (2020). Suicide, self-harm, & traumatic stress exposure: A trauma-informed approach to the evaluation and management of suicide risk. *Evidence-Based Practice in Child and Adolescent Mental Health, 5*(4), 483–500. https://doi.org/10.1080/23794925.2020.1796547

Bakken, V., Lydersen, S., Skokauskas, N., Sund, A. M., & Kaasbøll, J. (2024). Protective factors for suicidal ideation: A prospective study from adolescence to adulthood. *European Child & Adolescent Psychiatry.* https://doi.org/10.1007/s00787-024-02379-w

Barnhorst, A., Gonzales, H., & Asif-Sattar, R. (2021). Suicide prevention efforts in the United States and their effectiveness. *Current Opinion in Psychiatry, 34*(3), 299–305. https://doi.org/ 10.1097/YCO.0000000000000682

Barzilay, S., Yaseen, Z. S., Hawes, M., Gorman, B., Altman, R., Foster, A., Apter, A., Rosenfield, P., & Galynker, I. (2018). Emotional responses to suicidal patients: Factor structure, construct, and predictive validity of the Therapist Response Questionnaire-Suicide form. *Frontiers in Psychiatry, 9.* https://doi.org/10.3389/fpsyt.2018.00104

Bell, T. M., Qiao, N., Jenkins, P. C., Siedlecki, C. B., & Fecher, A. M. (2016). Trends in emergency department visits for nonfatal violence-related injuries among adolescents in the United States, 2009–2013. *The Journal of Adolescent Health: Official Publication of the Society for Adolescent Medicine, 58*(5), 573–575. https://doi.org/10.1016/j.jadohealth.2015.12.016

Bonanno, G. A. (2021). The resilience paradox. *European Journal of Psychotraumatology, 12*(1), 1942642. https://doi.org/10.1080/20008198.2021.1942642

Bonanno, G. A., Chen, S., Bagrodia, R., & Galatzer-Levy, I. R. (2024). Resilience and disaster: Flexible adaptation in the face of uncertain threat. *Annual Reviews, 75*, 573–599. https://doi.org/10.1146/annurev-psych-011123-024224

Brodsky, B. S., Spruch-Feiner, A., & Stanley, B. (2018). The zero suicide model: Applying evidence-based suicide prevention practices to clinical care. *Frontiers in Psychiatry, 9*, 33. https://doi.org/10.3389/fpsyt.2018.00033

Bryan, C. J., Mintz, J., Clemans, T. A., Leeson, B., Burch, T. S., Williams, S. R., Maney, E., & Rudd, M. D. (2017). Effect of crisis response planning vs. contracts for safety on suicide risk in U.S. Army Soldiers: A randomized clinical trial. *Journal of Affective Disorders, 212,* 64–72. https://doi.org/10.1016/j.jad.2017.01.028

Bühlmann, V., Schlüter-Müller, S., Fürer, L., Steppan, M., Birkhölzer, M., Schmeck, K., Koenig, J., Kaess, M., & Zimmermann, R. (2021). Therapists' emotional state after sessions in which suicidality is addressed: Need for improved management of suicidal tendencies in patients with borderline personality pathology. *BMC Psychiatry, 21*, 590. https://doi.org/10.1186/s12888-021-03549-9

Calo-Blanco, A., Kovářík, J., Mengel, F., & Romero, J. G. (2017). Natural disasters and indicators of social cohesion. *PloS One, 12*(6), 30176885. https://doi.org/10.1371/journal.pone.0176885

Caplan, G. (1961). *An approach to community mental health*. Grune and Stratton.

Caplan, G. (1964). *Principles of preventive psychiatry*. Basic Books.

Carr, M. J., Ashcroft, D. M., Kontopantelis, E., While, D., Awenat, Y., Cooper, J., Chew-Graham, C., Kapur, N., & Webb, R. T. (2017). Premature death among primary care patients with a history of self-harm. *Annals of Family Medicine, 15*(3), 246–254. https://doi.org/10.1370/afm.2054

Castellví, P., Lucas-Romero, E., Miranda-Mendizábal, A., Parés-Badell, O., Almenara, J., Alonso, I., Blasco, M. J., Cebrià, A., Gabilondo, A., Gili, M., Lagares, C., Piqueras, J. A., Roca, M., Rodríguez-Marín, T., Voto-Sanz, V., & Alonso, J. (2017). Longitudinal association between self-injurious thoughts and behaviors and suicidal behavior in adolescents and young adults: A systematic review with meta-analysis. *Journal of Affective Disorders, 215*, 37–48. https://doi.org/10.1016/j.jad.2017.03.035

Chaplin, S. (2023). NICE on the assessment and management of self-harm. *Prescriber, 34*(1), 21–22. https://doi.org/10.1002/psb.2033

Chen, J. I., Roth, B., Dobscha, S. K., & Lowery, J. C. (2024). Implementation strategies in suicide prevention: A scoping review. *Implementation Science, 19*, 20. https://doi.org/10.1186/s13012-024-1350-2

Curtin, S. C., & Heron, M. P. (2019). *Death rates due to suicide and homicide among persons aged 10–24: United States, 2000–2017*. Centers for Disease Control and Prevention. https://stacks.cdc.gov/view/cdc/81944

References

Dyregov, A., & Regel, S. (2012). Early interventions following exposure to traumatic events: Implications for practice from recent research. *Journal of Loss and Trauma, 17*(3), 271–291. https://doi.org/10.1080/15325024.2011.6168323

Edwards, S. J., & Sachmann, M. D. (2010). No-suicide contracts, no-suicide agreements, and no-suicide assurances: A study of their nature, utilization, perceived effectiveness, and potential to cause harm. *Crisis, 31*(6), 290–302. https://doi.org/10.1027/0227-5910/a000048

Feldman, R. (2020). What is resilience: An affiliative neuroscience approach. *World Psychiatry, 19*, 132–150. https://doi.org/10.1002/wps.20729

Franklin, J. C., Ribeiro, J. D., Fox, K. R., Bentley, K. H., Kleiman, E. M., Huang, X., Musacchio, K. M., Jaroszewski, A. C., Chang, B. P., & Nock, M. K. (2017). Risk factors for suicidal thoughts and behaviors: A meta-analysis of 50 years of research. *Psychological Bulletin, 143*(2), 187–232. https://doi.org/10.1037/bul0000084

Glenn, C. R., Kleiman, E. M., Kellerman, J., Pollak, O., Cha, C. B., Esposito, E. C., Porter, A. C., Wyman, P. A., & Boatman, A. E. (2020). Annual research review: A meta-analytic review of worldwide suicide rates in adolescents. *Journal of Child Psychology and Psychiatry, 61*(3), 294–308. https://doi.org/10.1111/jcpp.13106

Hedegaard, H., Curtin, S. C., & Warner, M. (2018). *Suicide mortality in the United States, 1999–2017*. https://www.cdc.gov/nchs/products/databriefs/db330.htm

Hermosilla, S., Forthal, S., Sadowska, K., Magill, E. B., Watson, P., & Pike, K. M. (2023). We need to build the evidence: A systematic review of psychological first aid on mental health and well-being. *Journal of Traumatic Stress, 36*(1), 5–16. https://doi.org/10.1002/jts.22888

Hobfoll, S. E., Watson, P., Bell, C. C., Bryant, R. A., Brymer, M. J., Friedman, M. J., Friedman, M., Gersons, B. P., de Jong, J. T., Layne, C. M., Maguen, S., Neria, Y., Norwood, A. E., Pynoos, R. S., Reissman, D., Ruzek, J. I., Shalev, A. Y., Solomon, Z., Steinberg, A. M., & Ursano, R. J. (2007). Five essential elements of immediate and mid-term mass trauma intervention: Empirical evidence. *Psychiatry, 70*(4), 283–369. https://doi.org/10.1521/psyc.2007.70.4.283

Horwitz, A. G., Czya, E. K., & King, C. A. (2014). Predicting future suicide attempts among adolescent and emerging adult psychiatric emergency patients. *Journal of Clinical Child and Adolescent Psychology: The Official Journal for the Society of Clinical Child and Adolescent Psychology, 44*(5), 751–761. https://doi.org/10.1080/15374416.2014.910789

Hughes, J. L., Ackerman, J. P., Adrian, M. C., Campo, J. V., & Bridge, J. A. (2023). Suicide in young people: Screening, risk assessment, and intervention. *British Medical Journal, 381*, e070630. https://doi.org/10.1136/bmj-2022-070630

James, R. K., & Gilliland, B. E. (2016). *Crisis intervention strategies* (8th ed.). Cengage.

Jones, N., Burdett, H., Green, K., & Greenberg, N. (2017). Trauma risk management (TRiM): Promoting help seeking for mental health problems among combat-exposed U.K. military personnel. *Psychiatry, 80*, 236–251. https://doi.org/10.1080/00332747.2017.1286894

Keyes, K. M., Kandula, S., Martinez-Ales, G., Gimbrone, C., Joseph, V., Monnat, S., Rutherford, C., Olfson, M., Gould, M., & Shaman, J. (2024). Geographic variation, economic activity, and labor market characteristics in trajectories of suicide in the United States, 2008–2020. *American Journal of Epidemiology, 193*(2), 256–266. https://doi.org/10.1093/aje/kwad205

King, C. A., Gipson Allen, P. Y., Ahamed, S. I., Webb, M., Casper, T. C., Brent, D., Grupp-Phelan, J., Rogers, T. A., Arango, A., Al-Dajani, N., McGuire, T. A., & Bagge, C. L. (2023). 24-hour warning signs for adolescent suicide attempts. *Psychological Medicine*, 1–12. https://doi.org/10.1017/S0033291723003112

Klonsky, E. D., Qiu, T. Y., & Saffer, B. Y. (2017). Recent advances in differentiating suicide attempters from suicide ideators. *Current Opinion in Psychiatry, 30*, 15–20. https://doi.org/10.1097.YCO.0000000000000294

Kusmaul, N. (2021). Role of trauma-informed care in disasters. In K. E. Cherry, & A. Gibson (Eds.), *The intersection of trauma and disaster behavioral health* (145–162). Springer. https://doi.org/10.1007/978-3-030-51525-6_9

Littlefield, A. K., Himes, K. P., Conner, K. R., & Bagge, C. L. (2024). Warning signs in a period of acute risk for suicide attempt: The utility of count- and combination-based classification. https://doi.org/10.2139/ssrn.4725809

Maslow, A. H. (1943). A theory of human motivation. *Psychological Review, 50*(4), 370–396. https://doi.org/10.1037/h0054346

Mehedi, N., & Ismail Hossain, M. (2022). Experiences of the frontline healthcare professionals amid the COVID-19 health hazard: A phenomenological investigation. *Inquiry: A Journal of Medical Care Organization, Provision and Financing, 59*, 1–11. https://doi.org/10.1177/00469580221111925

Meichenbaum, D. (1995). Disasters, stress and cognition. In S. E. Hobfoll & M. W. de Vries (Eds.), *Extreme stress and communities: Impact and intervention*. Springer. https://doi.org/10.1007/978-94-015-8486-9_2

Millner, A. J., Robinaugh, D. J., & Nock, M. K. (2020). Advancing the understanding of suicide: The need for formal theory and rigorous descriptive research. *Trends in Cognitive Sciences, 24*(9), 704–716. https://doi.org/10.1016/j.tics.2020.06.007

Mitchell, J. T. (1983). When disaster strikes – the critical incident stress debriefing process. *Journal of Emergency Medical Services, 8*, 36–39.

Mitchell, J. T., & Everly, G. S., Jr. (2023). Critical incident stress management (CISM). In M. L. Bourke, V. B. Van Hasselt, & S. J. Buser (Eds.), *First responder mental health* (pp. 179–209). Springer. https://doi.org/10.1007/978-3-031-38149-2_10

Mughal, F., Burton, F. M., Fletcher, H., Lascelle, K., O'Connor, R. C., Rae, S., Thomson, A. B., & Kapur, N. (2023). New guidance for self-harm: An opportunity not to be missed. *The British Journal of Psychiatry, 223*(5), 501–503. https://doi.org/10.1192/BJP.2023.113

References

National Guideline Alliance (U.K.). (2018). Evidence reviews for psychological, psychosocial and other non-pharmacological interventions for the prevention of PTSD in adults: Post-traumatic stress disorder: Evidence review. *National Institute for Health and Care Excellence* (NICE Guideline, No. 116). https://www.ncbi.nlm.nih.gov/books/NBK560223/

National Institute for Health and Care Excellence (NICE). (2022). Self-harm: Assessment, management and preventing recurrence. *NICE guideline*. www.nice.org.uk/guidance.ng225

Negri, A., Conte, F., Caldiroli, C. L., Neimeyer, R. A., & Castiglioni, M. (2023). Psychological factors explaining the COVID-19 pandemic impact on mental health: The role of meaning, beliefs, and perceptions of vulnerability and mortality. *Behavioral Sciences*, *13*(2), 162. https://doi.org/10.3390/bs13020162

O'Connor, R. C., & Portzky, G. (2018). The relationship between entrapment and suicidal behavior through the lens of the integrated motivational–volitional model of suicidal behavior. *Current Opinion in Psychology*, *22*, 12–17. https://doi.org/10.1016/j.copsyc.2017.07.021

Pathirathna, M., Nandasena, H. M. R. K. G., Atapattu, A. M. M. P., & Weerasekara, I. (2022). Impact of the COVID-19 pandemic on suicidal attempts and death rates: A systematic review. *BMC Psychiatry*, *22*, 506. https://doi.org/10.1186/s12888-022-04158-w

Pau, K., Ahnad, A., & Tang, H. Y. (2020). Crisis, disaster, and trauma counseling: Implications for the counseling profession. *Journal of Critical Reviews*, *7*(8), 736–739. https://doi.org/10.31838/jcr.07.08.160

Picoult, J. (2004). *My sister's keeper*. Atria.

Quinlivan, L., Gorman, L., Littlewood, D. L., Monaghan, E., Barlow, S. J., Campbell, S., Webb, R. T., & Kapur, N. (2022). 'Wasn't offered one, too poorly to ask for one'—Reasons why some patients do not receive a psychosocial assessment following self-harm: Qualitative patient and carer survey. *Australian & New Zealand Journal of Psychiatry*, *56*(4), 398–407. https://doi.org/10.1177/00048674211011262

Quinn, T., Adger, W. N., Butler, C., & Walker-Springett, K. (2021). Community resilience and well-being: An exploration of relationality and belonging after disasters. *Annals of the American Association of Geographers*, *111*(2), 577–590. https://doi.org/10.1080/24694452.2020.1782167

Richins, M. T., Gauntlett, L., Tehrani, N., Hesketh, I., Weston, D., Carter, H., & Amlôt, R. (2020). Early post-trauma interventions in organizations: A scoping review. *Frontiers in Psychology*, *11*, 1176. https://doi.org/10.3389/fpsyg.2020.01176

Rico, E. (2016). *Teaching and evaluation of suicidal assessment: Five-step evaluation and triage (SAFE-T)*. California State University.

Roberts, A. R., & Ottens, A. J. (2005). The seven-stage crisis intervention model: A road map to goal attainment, problem solving, and crisis resolution. *Brief Treatment and Crisis Intervention*, *5*(4), 329–339. https://doi.org/10.1093/brief-treatment/mhi030

Rosenberg, H., Errett, N. A., & Eisenman, D. P. (2022). Working with disaster-affected communities to envision healthier futures: A trauma-informed approach to post-disaster recovery planning. *International Journal of Environmental Research and Public Health, 19*(3), 1723. https://doi.org/10.3390/ijerph19031723

Rozek, D. C., & Bryan, C. J. (2020). Integrating crisis response planning for suicide prevention into trauma-focused treatments: A military case example. *Journal of Clinical Psychology, 76*(5), 852–864. https://doi.org/10.1002/jclp.22920

Rudd, M. D., Berman, A. L., Joiner, T. E., Nock, M. K., Silverman, M. M., Mandrusiak, M., Van Orden, K., & Witte, T. (2006). Warning signs for suicide: Theory, research, and clinical applications. *Suicide and Life-Threatening Behavior, 36*(3), 255–262. https://doi.org/10.1521/suli.2006.36.3.255

Saunders, K. R. K., McGuinness, E., Barnett, P., Foye, U., Sears, J., Carlisle, S., Allman, F., Tzouvara, V., Schlief, M., San Juan, N. V., Stuart, R., Griffiths, J., Appleton, R., McCrone, P., Olive, R. R., Nyikavaranda, P., Jeynes, T., Mitchell, L., Simpson, A., Johnson, S., & Trevillion, K. (2023). A scoping review of trauma-informed approaches in acute, crisis, emergency, and residential mental health care. *BMC Psychiatry, 23*, 567. https://doi.org/10.1186/s12888-023-05016-a

Scott, Z., O'Curry, S., & Mastroyannopoulou, K. (2022). The impact and experience of debriefing for clinical staff following traumatic events in clinical settings: A systematic review. *Journal of Traumatic Stress, 35*(1), 278–287. https://doi.org/10.1002/jts.22736

Slone, H., Gutierrez, A., Lutzky, C., Zhu, D., Hedriana, H., Barrera, J. F., Paige, S. R., & Bunnell, B. E. (2021). Assessing the impact of COVID-19 on mental health providers in the southeastern United States. *Psychiatry Research, 302*, 114055. https://doi.org/10.1016/j.psychres.2021.114055

Substance Abuse and Mental Health Services Administration (SAMHSA). (2014). *SAMHSA's concept of trauma and guidance for a trauma-informed approach* [pdf file]. Substance Abuse and Mental Health Services Administration.

Tsai, M., & Klonsky, E. D. (2023). Warning signs for suicide attempts in psychiatric inpatients: Patient and informant perspectives. *General Hospital Psychiatry, 85*, 207–212. https://doi.org/10.1016/j.genhosppsych.2023.11.005

Uddin, T., Pitman, A., Benson, G., Kamal, Z., Hawton, K., & Rowe, S. (2023). Attitudes toward and experiences of clinical and non-clinical services among individuals who self-harm or attempt suicide: A systematic review. *Psychological Medicine, 54*(1), 13–31. https://doi.org/10.1017/S0033291723002805

Van Orden, K. A., Witte, T. K., Gordon, K. H., Bender, T. W., & Joiner, T. E., Jr. (2008). Suicidal desire and the capability for suicide: Tests of the interpersonal-psychological theory of suicidal behavior among adults. *Journal of Consulting and Clinical Psychology, 76*(1), 72–83. https://doi.org/10.1037/0022-006X.76.1.72

Varshney, K., Patel, H., & Panhwar, M. A. (2024). Risks and warning signs for medical student suicide mortality: A systematic review. *Archives of Suicide Research*. https://doi.org/10.1080/13811118.2024.2310553

Walker, B. H. (2020). Resilience: What it *is* and is *not*. *Ecology & Society*, *25*(2), 11. https://doi.org/10.5751/ES-11647-250211

Wang, L., Norman, I., Xiao, T., Li, Y., & Leamy, M. (2021). Psychological first aid training: A scoping review of its application, outcomes and implementation. *International Journal of Environmental Research and Public Health*, 18(9), 4594. https://doi.org/10.3390/ijerph18094594

Watson, L., & Andrews, L. (2018). The effect of a Trauma Risk Management (TRiM) program on stigma and barriers to help-seeking in the police. *International Journal of Stress Management*, *25*(4), 348–356. https://doi.org/10.1037/str0000071

Westers, N. J., & Plener, P. L. (2020). Managing risk and self-harm: Keeping young people safe. *Clinical Child Psychology and Psychiatry*, *24*(3). https://doi.org/10.1177/1359104519895064

Xiao, Y., Junus, A., Li, T., & Yip, P. (2023). Temporal and spatial trends in suicide-related visits before and during the COVID-19 pandemic in the U.S., 2018–2021. *Journal of Affective Disorders*, *324*, 24–35. https://doi.org/10.1016/j.jad.2022.12.062

Zortea, T. C., Cleare, S., Melson, A. J., Wetherall, K., & O'Connor, R. C. (2020). Understanding and managing suicide risk. *British Medical Bulletin*, *134*, 73–84. https://doi.org/10.1093/bmb/ldaa013

Chapter Eight
Challenges in Trauma Work

Overview

Trauma and crisis counseling is rewarding work. However, challenges arise for professionals who want to help trauma survivors. Chapter 8, Challenges in Trauma Work, discusses the obstacles in treating trauma related to systems, clients, and clinicians. Working ethically, trauma workers should consider their professional motivation, the systemic challenges, the issues related to different client populations, and the barriers for clients and clinicians to ensure the best possible outcomes. The chapter explores the application of ethical principles to trauma-informed care. Maintaining a perspective on client and counselor resilience is possible despite the challenges.

Harder than You Think

As we teach and speak at conferences and workshops or engage in casual conversation about trauma work, we notice several assumptions arise. One reason is curiosity about the intensity of counseling and its similarity to other psychotherapy treatments. These assumptions convey the fundamental beliefs about trauma: it demands effort and entails similar types of work. We respond that counseling traumatized clients is harder than you think, unlike the psychotherapy we do with other clients. The difference in trauma work may be best described as a circuitous route through mountains and valleys, often leading to unknown roads. It is not a horizontal superhighway from beginning to end.

DOI: 10.4324/9781003463009-8

The World Health Organization surveyed 70,000 adults from 24 countries and identified that 70.4% of those individuals had experienced at least one trauma at some point (Wathen et al., 2023). However, some do not receive the help they need because of the challenges in trauma work. While professionals want to help traumatized people, they face obstacles related to systems, clients, and clinicians. As discussed in previous chapters, the neglect to care for clients with trauma may be because of the lack of clarity about the terms used in the trauma field, the scarcity of research on measurements, understudied socio-ecological levels, the components for treatment, and the treatment contexts (Champine et al., 2019). It may also be because some people experience a traumatic event and have symptoms but do not meet the criteria for PTSD. This situation can lead to further victimization or stigmatization of those people (Fernández et al., 2023). As a result, being informed about trauma is crucial for organizations and professional workers. To address the challenges in trauma work means trauma workers should weigh the benefits with their ethical motivation, the systemic challenges, the issues related to different client populations, and the barriers for clinicians.

Ethical Considerations

If you work as a licensed professional counselor, you cannot avoid clients with trauma. While thrust into such work, one may not be prepared or desire to be a trauma professional. To engage in the work with the best possible outcomes, a therapist should consider their professional motivation, review the ethical principles, and understand the challenges of trauma work. Challenges in trauma work are plentiful, and, often, clients can present complex problems that may lead to ethical principles that conflict (Welfel, 2016). Ethical dilemmas can feel overwhelming to those new to helping traumatized individuals. In graduate programs, we instruct future practitioners to consult and document, and we must remember that the client will also often feel emotional distress in such situations.

Motivation

A relevant question for anyone who desires to work with traumatized individuals becomes, "Why do I want to do this work?" Examining one's motivation is a crucial factor and may predict success with clients who experience trauma. When engaging in trauma work, a good question is, "Whose need does this meet?" Self-reflection and self-supervision are essential skills. If the goal is because you have experienced trauma, the next question becomes, "What have you done to resolve your primary trauma?" Approximately 30% of mental health professionals report some trauma history. A personal experience with trauma predisposes one to secondary trauma (Leung et al., 2023). However, some studies show trauma survivors prefer working with others who have related experiences. They feel more supported, believed, and respected (Konya et al., 2020; Robotham et al., 2019). While some may enter the field with a desire to help trauma survivors because they are also survivors, that motivation may or may not be sufficient.

Some people are motivated to help others because they care about people. Despite this altruism, it can increase the risk of compassion fatigue for the professional or non-professional worker. Figley addresses this in his model of compassion fatigue when he refers to how empathic concern and response can lead to compassion fatigue if not mitigated by compassion satisfaction (Figley, 2002). This discussion leads to the question one should be asking, "What is the best motivation for working in the trauma field? Is there a good reason to do this work? The answer to the first is "Because people have a need, and I trained to do this work," and the response to the latter is "Absolutely." Having the right motivation will benefit the client and the therapist more.

Nurture Understanding

- What might be insufficient reasons as you think about motivation for helping people with trauma?
- What type of motivation do you believe is most important in choosing to work with trauma survivors?

Ethical Principles

When we speak of ethical principles, we are talking about values, how the clinician uses or interprets those values, how those apply in practice, and how we honor the values of the person we treat. These values or principles may vary according to individuals, groups, or cultures. Most professions have a code of ethics guiding actions and responses as they seek to provide services to others. These codes of ethics protect the profession, provide a core set of conditions for the profession, and protect the professionals (Anriani et al., 2022). The code of ethics sets the expectations and standards, thus ensuring consumers that consistency in practice is valued and that

Ethical Considerations

a minimal expectation for moral behavior is provided (Aulia et al., 2024). Codes of ethics exist for psychologists, professional counselors, licensed marriage and family therapists, and other counseling professionals. The licensing boards of these professions determine the code of ethics, and individuals who desire licensure must know and agree to follow this code.

These codes also aid professional counselors in making decisions. However, sometimes, codes conflict or ambiguous situations surface (Cottone et al., 2021; Johnson et al., 2022). These present ethical dilemmas wherein a counselor must choose which principle takes precedence. To do so in a professional manner may involve consultation with professional peers or legal advocates. Another consideration about ethical codes is the disagreements in ethical issues surrounding the counseling relationship and boundaries, confidentiality, cultural values, professional responsibility, and technology. The sociopolitical climate influence how these are interpreted by case law (Carlisle et al., 2022).

In general, the ethics codes identify primary principles that serve as a foundation for counseling. These include autonomy, justice, beneficence, nonmaleficence, and fidelity (Forester-Miller & Davis, 2016). Providing autonomy in trauma-informed care means respecting the trauma survivor's need for independence and determination of what they desire in treatment. This freedom allows the client to make decisions based on their values. To offer this, clinicians must inform the client about their treatment options while assessing the individual's ability to make such decisions (Forester-Miller & Davis, 2016). Informed consent incorporates the client's ability to understand the information necessary to decide and the ramifications of their choice. Trauma-informed care means offering information with transparency, providing individuals with reasonable expectations, and a plan for recourse or grievance, if needed. Finally, informed consent must be voluntary (Lin et al., 2019). For example, a therapist should inform a client of the possible advantages and disadvantages of therapeutic techniques, even technology-assisted tools. To request that a client use a software application without explaining that providing their information to download the tool may cause a breach of confidentiality is unethical.

In applying justice, the therapist offers counseling appropriate to the individual, given their abilities, cultural background, and needs. It does not mean treating everyone equally but according to their needs (Kitchener & Anderson, 2011). Therapists employ justice when they acknowledge the role of intergenerational, historical, and institutional trauma and when they are sensitive to minority stress or that which occurs because of micro-aggressions, racism, violence, or hatred perpetrated against a minority group. It means adjusting one's approach according to the needs and history of the client and maintaining an awareness of one's words and actions that can continue to traumatize the individual (Stark et al., 2022). An example would be applying the exact expectations, fundamental understanding, or approaches to clients of different ethnicities or cultural backgrounds.

The principle of beneficence is doing good and being proactive, while nonmaleficence means not causing harm to another person. In applying both, the clinician must be sensitive to the use of assessment tools, diagnostic considerations, and the application of approaches (Rizvi et al., 2021). Many helpers want to do something helpful for the traumatized individual. Doing good means providing a safe environment for the client, including therapy interactions. Providing beneficence means setting appropriate boundaries and being mindful of self-disclosure and how these might be beneficial or harmful to the individual. It also means the therapist is aware when countertransference occurs in therapy (Jenks & Oka, 2022). Nonmaleficence means avoiding intentional harm or saying or doing things that may cause harm (Kitchener, 1984). This principle means discussing with a client the potential benefits and risks of all treatment interventions (Jenks & Oka, 2022). Welfel (2016) posits that nonmaleficence is the most essential principle and takes priority over all other principles.

Finally, fidelity means being loyal, faithful, and honoring commitments to the client. Having fidelity is related to the counselor's adherence to treatment standards and best practices, level of competency or skill, and treatment differentiation (Holder et al., 2018). In other words, do you practice counseling at the highest standard of care, are you competent to treat traumatized individuals, and do you offer approaches based on their greatest need? Do you deliver what you have offered to the client? The promise of care for a client rests on the commitment of the therapist to offer their time and effort while remaining true to the protocol they implement. If a different approach is needed, then fidelity means discussing a change in therapy with the client.

Ethical Challenges

One will encounter ethical challenges in counseling. The most common issues in the counseling relationship are confidentiality and privacy issues, group work, termination and referral, and distance counseling. While these lead to ethical dilemmas, most challenges are systemic issues, client factors, and clinician concerns and practices. Counselors must respond with care, patience, and wisdom when ethical challenges come. The steps in proceeding with the case should include critical reflection about the case, reviewing the available information, identifying the possible options, consulting with a professional peer or supervisor, reviewing your ethics code, determining which ethical principles are at stake, identifying any legal issues or agency policy violations, identifying a course of action, implementing, and documenting the process, and post-reflection (Kitchener & Anderson, 2011).

The influence of consultations can aid practitioners in motivation, self-efficacy, and more robust decision-making. Consultation is typical, especially in complex cases (Cook et al., 2019). As graduate programs strive to develop ethical practitioners, we see that real-life therapeutic circumstances make applying codes and principles distressing. More consistent training or understanding of the need for ongoing consultation beyond licensure requirements is needed (Cook et al., 2019) (Figure 8.1).

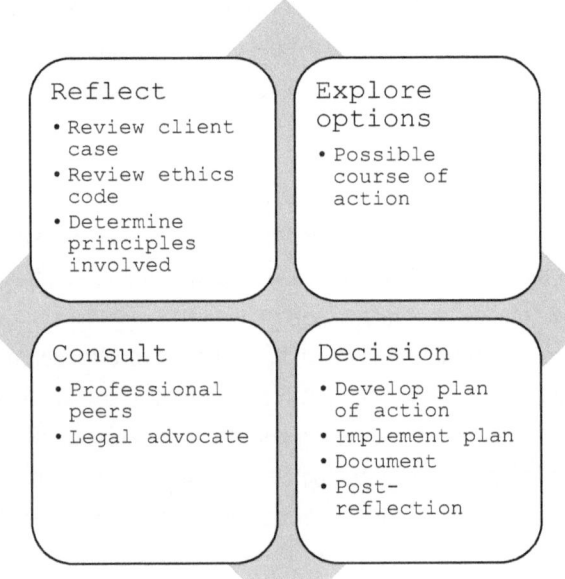

FIGURE 8.1 How to Process Ethical Dilemmas.

(Adapted from Kitchener & Anderson, 2011; Cook et al., 2019).

Cultivate Knowledge

As you consider the ethical principles of autonomy, justice, beneficence, nonmalefi-cence, and fidelity, review this fictional case and follow the steps to determine an action plan.

Trevor has completed six sessions of therapy with you. His insurance plan will not cover further sessions, and Trevor states he cannot afford further sessions. Trevor's history of trauma is of concern because of the ongoing physical abuse during child-hood from his father and his mother's tendency to control and manipulate him. In addition, Trevor has recently ended a relationship in which he was physically and emotionally abused by his partner. When Trevor started therapy, he and you thought getting more therapy sessions from his third-party payor would likely occur. Trevor has made progress in self-regulation skills. However, his symptoms of over-reactivity, cog-nitive distortions, and shame are not resolved. Trevor needs further help and he asks if you will continue to see him at a significantly reduced rate. This concern presents an ethical dilemma for you:

1. What is your initial response to Trevor? What are the possible implications? What internal reaction do you have?
2. Review Trevor's history and progress; what are your thoughts?
3. What are the possible options for Trevor's treatment?
4. What does your ethics code say about treatment? Refer to the ACA 2014 Code of Ethics for this question.
5. What ethical principles are essential? Are any principles in conflict with one another?
6. What legal issues are present? With whom would you consult?
7. What action plan will you take?

Facing the Barriers

When a trauma survivor desires to recover, there are a myriad of barriers they might face. It can be like walking through a maze where one enters a walkway, taking twists and turns, only to discover a dead end. When a person faces enough of these barri-ers, their motivation for recovery may diminish, they will become frustrated, or their lack of trust in the mental health system will fade. These barriers may be the result of

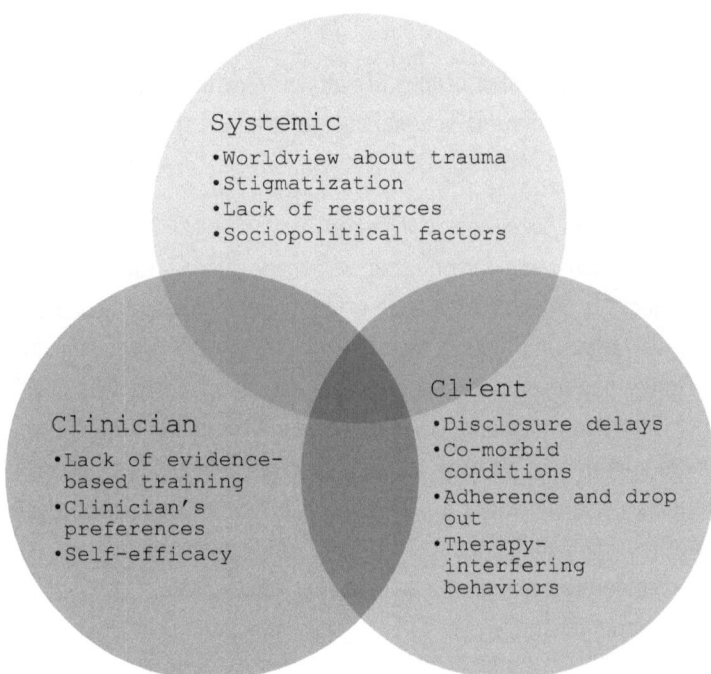

FIGURE 8.2 Challenges or Barriers in Trauma Work.

(Adapted from De Boer et al., 2022; Lashkay et al., 2023; Mueller et al., 2008; Wagner et al., 2012).

how systems, society, clients, and clinicians view and manage trauma and the use of interventions (Figure 8.2).

Systemic Challenges

While we like to think we have a caring society, some challenges appear when trauma occurs. Indeed, our society is more open than ever before to receiving psychotherapeutic help. However, some still have an implicit bias toward those who need or seek mental health services. This partiality is apparent in the inadequate healthcare policies in organizations throughout the U.S. (Kazlauskas, 2017). There is still stigmatization that traumatized individuals face. This stigma appears in the casual comments that some people make about traumatized people, minority groups, or individuals who need continuing support (De Boer et al., 2022; Lashkay et al., 2023; Mueller et al., 2008; Wagner et al., 2012).

Combine the above elements with socioeconomic factors, including those populations with less access to quality healthcare and in lower income brackets, the lack of resources available to specific populations, and the limited training of medical providers (Finch et al., 2020; Hoysted et al., 2018; Kazlauskas, 2017). This factor means that agencies or providers may not inquire about patients' trauma or offer screening. Disagreement about screening, screening tools, and the process becomes a barrier (Evaldas, 2017; Menschner & Maul, 2016). Even when organizations do screen, these are quick screens that may occur without a thorough psychosocial assessment. This inadequate screening may be because of time limitations, access to screening instruments, or education (Hoysted et al., 2018).

Finally, access to training and resources and the dissemination of treatment approaches may be a barrier because of the time and cost of receiving these. With a shortage of mental health providers in the nation, clinician caseloads are full, offering little time to complete an entire course in trauma (U.S. Government Accountability Office, 2024). There are difficulties related to finding trauma-informed therapists in specific geographic locations where internet access is limited (Ferrell et al., 2019). These issues related to stigmatization, power, socioeconomics, and access are relevant, and communities and states must address them. However, there are also barriers related to clients and clinicians. Therefore, a multi-prong approach is required.

Client Challenges

Clients present with unique challenges. The first is a trauma survivor's avoidance of trauma disclosure. This avoidance is symptomatic of trauma and is a significant predictor of PTSD (Kantor et al., 2017; Kazlauskas, 2017). Numerous adults who experience childhood abuse do not disclose for at least five years after the first occurrence of abuse, with the average delay of disclosure at 21 years (McElvaney, 2015; Tener & Murphy, 2015). The reasons for the delay are intrapersonal, interpersonal, and sociocultural. Clients often experience shame or guilt about abuse, doubting their perception of the event(s) or the accuracy of their memory. They may fear the reaction of their friends, families, loved ones, or anyone who hears their story. The fear of how disclosure will impact their lives, jobs, and social interactions is prevalent (Tener & Murphy, 2015). This lack of disclosure means clients will not receive the referrals, recommendations, or treatment they may need. Because clients seek someone trustworthy, the therapeutic alliance is crucial.

Another challenge with clients is the comorbidity of conditions discussed in Chapter 5: Diagnosing Trauma. Aside from depressive, anxiety, or personality disorders, clients may have other conditions that delay or complicate treatment. These may include

Facing the Barriers

learning disabilities, developmental delays, struggles with hearing or deafness, processing disorders, or neurodiverse individuals (Finch et al., 2020). The field of traumatology is just entering the era where targeted treatments for such populations or conditions are developing.

Client treatment adherence and early dropout of therapy are problematic. Adults and children drop out of treatment prematurely. In evidence-based treatments for PTSD, the dropout rate for adults was between 18 and 72% (DeViva, 2014; Kehle-Forbes et al., 2016; Mott et al., 2014). Even in Cognitive Processing Therapy, dropout rates are significant (Sijercic et al., 2021). Other studies indicate a high dropout rate among children and adolescents (Skar et al., 2022). When treatment adherence is compromised, clients do not receive the total dosage. This occurrence is akin to taking half of a prescription for an antibiotic, which proves unsuccessful at resolving the problem.

There are times when clients engage in therapy-interfering behaviors. These may be avoidance behaviors such as canceling appointments, arriving late, not showing up for scheduled appointments, and engaging in light conversation for most of the therapy hour. Other therapy-interfering behaviors might include ongoing suicidal ideation or gestures. Some clients will not complete homework assignments. Reducing therapy-interfering behaviors can increase the client's completion of therapy (May et al., 2016). There are strategies to help with these behaviors, but the key is exploring the rationale for these and addressing the client's avoidance of trauma material. Clinicians must provide extensive skills training for clients to address escape behaviors and increase distress tolerance (Brown & Dahlin, 2017). In addition, the therapist's validation of the client's suffering, which is the root of therapy-interfering behaviors, needs to be the priority. As the therapeutic alliance strengthens, the client will develop trust, and the behaviors can be changed (Yang et al., 2017).

Clinician Challenges

While there are systemic barriers and client challenges, further problems occur that are related to the trauma helper. While these are usually unintentional, they can have a profound effect on a traumatized person who struggles with attachment and trust. These include the lack of training in trauma, the clinician's preferences, and the therapist's self-efficacy.

Throughout this text, we discuss the lack of training in trauma. While many clinicians purchase books and materials to help, and others attend workshops, few engage in ongoing peer supervision or consultation in treating trauma that evidence-based program certifications require. While therapists attempt to find the missing education, there remains too little use of evidence-based practices (Wathen et al., 2023). In a national survey of therapists working with clients who have eating disorders, familiarity with evidence-based practices in trauma was low (Trottier et al., 2017). In a meta-analysis of licensed therapists, the reasons for the lack of use of evidence-based practices were the view that the intervention manuals were too rigid, the difficulty adapting to a group-based approach, an inflexible treatment length, the lack of guideline flexibility, and the ability to adapt the approach to meet an individual client's need (Finch et al., 2020). This lack of understanding speaks to a need for further deployment of education regarding evidence-based practices and clinicians managing the ambiguity that comes with applying practices to clients (Brown & Courtois, 2019).

As one begins to practice counseling, they develop a style, gather resources, and acquire interventions that fit their role and clientele. This practice becomes a comfortable space for clinicians. Licensed professionals are required to complete continuing education to maintain licensure. Additional courses in therapeutic applications are widespread. However, therapists want to apply what they have learned to fit their context. This practice means they might pick and choose the components they wish to apply. The avoidance of evidence-based practices is due, in part, to the clinician's perception that they must follow the manualized approach (Marques et al., 2016). However, there is a need for clarification with these approaches. It is possible to remain faithful to the protocol and be flexible in its application. This view relies on the therapist's understanding of the primary treatment framework and theories used (Finch et al., 2020).

Another aspect related to clinician preference is the view that trauma work is time-intensive (Kirst et al., 2017) and may not be what the client desires. Evidence-based treatments aim at reducing posttraumatic stress symptoms, but, often, clients' expectations of therapy include self-respect, improved functioning, and enhanced social relationships (Gnaulati, 2019). Therapists must balance clients' desires with third-party payors and other stakeholders' requests. Trauma-focused therapy needs a minimum of 9–20 sessions of weekly therapy for 50% of clients to show clinically significant change (Lambert et al., 2001). The therapist must work hard to sustain the client for at least

Facing the Barriers

six months to achieve positive results while preventing dropout. While training and perception matter, another challenge for clinicians is their self-confidence.

In working with trauma, clinicians tend to feel less confident. They believe they lack competence and experience (Finch et al., 2020). A sense of self-efficacy is crucial in treating trauma survivors. Self-efficacy is the helper's perception of their ability to provide effective treatment and is a motivational force in using evidence-based practices (LoParo et al., 2019; Shapiro et al., 2021). The therapist's perception of competence in an evidence-based practice like TF-CBT is a significant predictor of posttraumatic stress treatment response (Espeleta et al., 2022). This lack of confidence creates uncertainty for the clinician, who questions when and how to implement interventions and determine which are in the patient's best interest (Yang et al., 2017). Decreased self-efficacy is related to less trauma screening and the lack of attention to trauma in clients (Salyers et al., 2004). However, higher self-efficacy is associated with less burnout and less emotional exhaustion (Finkstein et al., 2015; Kim et al., 2018).

Maintaining healthy boundaries in the counseling relationship requires increased self-efficacy. When working with trauma survivors, you can feel like they should be given greater latitude in boundaries because of their traumatic history. Boundary crossing may occur, such as attending a client event outside the therapy session. While your intention may be kindhearted, how a client perceives this may differ. This violation can create problems and prevent progress (Oramas, 2017). The concept of boundaries is providing a protective frame for the client. It refers to appropriate behavior in a therapeutic context that applies to the relationship's physical, psychological, and social aspects (Gutheil & Brodsky, 2008). Boundary violations may include therapist self-disclosure or inappropriate touch (Blundell et al., 2022). There is disagreement among ethicists about therapist self-disclosure, as some clients prefer therapists who share their experiences with trauma (Jolley, 2019). A counselor with questions about boundaries should use peer consultation or supervision.

Tending Your Technique

Determining appropriate boundaries is difficult in working with trauma survivors:

- What types of boundaries do you think are most important in working with clients who have experienced trauma?

- In what ways can you demonstrate care and concern with a traumatized client while setting boundaries?
- How would you respond if a client asks to be your friend on social media?

Moving to Solutions

While challenges exist, we need to explore the possible solutions. Interestingly, the solutions fit together like a puzzle, each affecting the other. We are reminded of the game we played with dominoes growing up. As children, we stood those on end, close together, and created a line with dominoes. Then we knocked one down, and they all tipped over. The issues present in treating trauma are related, albeit complex. However, we can overcome them together.

Systemic Solutions

The systemic issues that currently exist are related to sociopolitical forces. The division of political allegiances and conflicts arises from differing worldviews. Sire (2020) posits that all worldviews must answer specific questions about prime reality, world nature, human beings, epistemology, ethics, and meaning. What is your foundation, the fundamental belief, that provides you strength, hope, and courage? How do you view the world around you? Do you view it as a wonderful, creative, connected place or a dismal, hopeless one? What do you believe about clients with trauma histories? Are they creative, resourceful, and whole, or are they manipulative? How do you know what is truth? Is there one way to view things? What principles guide your actions in society? What is the meaning of your life, your community, and your nation? The answers to these questions inform how you treat others, live your life, and what you are willing to do to create systemic change.

Changing worldviews, or our perspective about a specific issue, means considering other viewpoints, methods, and ideas. Consider what might happen if we consistently adopt a salutogenic approach to psychological health. In this view, we might research the protective factors and the fundamental causes of trauma and then identify what needs to change on a community, state, and national level. We could explore how structures cause suffering and shift to those that create healing (Siddique, 2018). Offering trauma-informed care leads to increased satisfaction for an individual and the system (Carter & Blanch, 2019). Changing means everyone understands that trauma is not an individual issue but a social problem that requires improving care delivery or how we provide novel programs that value patients, staff, and care providers and place persons above profit (Siddique, 2018).

Addressing the challenges that exist in systems requires that we reduce the stigmatization of trauma survivors and the discriminatory practices that perpetuate victimization and stereotypes (Quinn et al., 2014). When traumatized individuals experience such judgment, they internalize it, which exacerbates their posttraumatic stress symptoms (Banaj & Pellicano, 2020). Re-traumatization means that trauma survivors may have a more challenging time functioning at their best, and this affects how they interact at a systems level. Changing stigma means believing a person's story instead of doubting its veracity. It means shifting from blame to offering hope and help. Finally, it means providing the support and resources most needed (Delker et al., 2020). This change begins with you as you examine your initial reactions to people in public places who seem displaced. As we increase our awareness that these people may be wounded, we can offer aid instead of judgment and a calming presence of safety to help them find more effective ways to express their needs and tell their stories. It is the expression of describing what happened in a context of trust that survivors begin to understand who they are and can build a coherent self (Delker et al., 2020).

Meeting Client Challenges

While we work to bring systemic change, consider how those influence clients. If a trauma survivor can find a trustworthy person with knowledge and experience, they can disclose sooner. The potential healing occurs when helpers understand trauma and how it relates to the individual's current behaviors, thoughts, and difficulties. Unfortunately, clients seek assistance but find it unhelpful when therapists do not ask about trauma, are uninterested in how it affects them currently, or ask too many details too quickly (Knight, 2019). As we teach and offer workshops, too often, people remark they attended a few therapy sessions wherein the therapist told them they needed to go for counseling elsewhere if they have a trauma history. Trauma survivors see this as rejection and disbelief in their story.

People may have several diagnoses, including PTSD, depression, or other conditions. These case presentations can be challenging for the novice counselor. However, part of being a professional helper is advancing practice skills, learning evidence-based methods, and gaining competency in treating such conditions. We are proud when our licensure candidates carefully prepare for their clients by attending seminars, reading research, and practicing skills. Thus, doing so enhances the counseling process for the client and allows exploration of the reciprocal nature of comorbid conditions.

When clients display therapy-interfering behaviors, it is best to explore why these exist instead of using punitive measures (Brissett et al., 2023). There are times when it takes great effort for a client to show up for an appointment. Clients struggle with pain, and this leads to suicidal thinking or non-suicidal self-injury. It is not a ploy to seek attention but rather a cry for help, "I don't know how I can continue to bear so much hurt." The therapist's sensitivity and response to the client can be a turning point. While one may think they can remain neutral, every word and action of a thera- pist has a connotation (Yang et al., 2017). The best response is to affirm the client's need for help. While the temptation is to correct the client or improve their actions or thoughts when clients use therapy-interfering behaviors, the wise trauma helper focuses on what is happening rather than what is wrong (Gnaulati, 2019). When we see these therapy-interfering behaviors as survival skills, then we become more help- ful (Levenson, 2017). It may be that a client is re-enacting their trauma, so these instances provide opportunities to explore the trauma (Knight, 2019).

To increase treatment adherence and decrease dropout rates, the therapist must understand the most common reasons their patients do so. Some drop out because they have concerns about how long recovery will take and how it will change their future. Others are ambivalent about receiving therapy, how it will look, and whether it will work. Others do so because of the surrounding stigma or natural barriers that arrive, including limited financial resources, lack of time availability, and other com- mitments. Clients remain in treatment when they see progress, receive encourage- ment from significant others, have a supportive relationship with a therapist, and have a desire to believe that therapy helps (Gjerstad et al., 2024). In a qualitative study with veterans, the dropout rate was correlated to the patient's interpretation of their symp- toms and practical barriers. If they felt therapy was not working or that treatment was interfering with their functioning, then they decided to leave (Kehle-Forbes et al., 2022). Anticipatory concerns, such as therapy making things worse, contributed to early dropout. Things that changed their perception of treatment efficacy were having new insights, success in moving past points where they were stuck, and self- regulation skills (Alpert et al., 2024). The solution may come when therapists discuss

Moving to Solutions

client expectations for therapy and the recovery process in the initial sessions. However, these suggestions are reliant upon clinician factors.

Changes for Clinicians

When survivors of trauma seek help, they look for providers with training and experience. These factors coincide with therapists' self-efficacy. Additional training increases counselor self-efficacy, including confidence and skill (Shapiro et al., 2021). If therapists do not receive training in evidence-based trauma therapies, they tend to have lower self-efficacy and avoid treating trauma cases (Finch et al., 2020). Being trained in more than one trauma-focused approach also increases self-efficacy. In-person workshops, clinical supervision, and peer consultation also correlate with higher self-efficacy (Becker-Haimes et al., 2022; Kerns et al., 2016). Combining training, supervision, or consultation and increasing skill practice enhances the therapeutic relationship.

As one can see, these barriers in treatment can be addressed in singular ways and yet have a synergistic effect on the whole of the challenges. Making the changes needed does require commitment, time, and energy. Once a therapist sees the benefits and how it protects them as professionals, they may be more willing to invest in making the modifications.

Gather Self-Awareness

Answer the following questions:

- What are your thoughts about the systemic changes that need to occur? What is your role in making that happen?
- Do you have other solutions for client challenges? Describe those.
- In what ways can you build your self-efficacy as a trauma worker?

A Flourishing Focus

Trauma and crisis counseling provide several benefits. Therapists working in nonprofit organizations feel a sense of reward and a deepening of their sense of humanity.

Caring and empathy are rewarding experiences (Melaki & Stavrou, 2023). This feeling of achievement is often described as compassion satisfaction, which is the positive feelings that arise from helping others (Stamm, 1995). There is a positive correlation between compassion satisfaction and resilience (Unjai et al., 2022). Therapists working in private practice experience an increasing appreciation for humanity and an improved sense of well-being. Doing this trauma work also increases one's satisfaction and depth of appreciation for life (Melaki & Stavrou, 2023).

In a qualitative study, therapists identified being called or drawn to the work of trauma while feeling a deep connection and oneness with the survivor. The trauma worker could maintain a sense of separateness while leading the trauma victim "out of the darkness" (Coleman et al., 2018, p. 2801). Stamm (1995) refers to compassion satisfaction, the sense of strength and meaning one gains when helping another person in the healing process. Figley notes that compassion satisfaction is a protective factor that mitigates the deleterious effects of compassion stress, preventing secondary trauma (Figley, 2002). The best part is helping people find meaning and a sense of purpose that propels them into a new life. That is posttraumatic growth (Coleman et al., 2018). To do so requires a healthy presence, and with that comes self-confidence, sensitivity, compassion, and deepening sensitivity (Ali et al., 2023).

The reward and satisfaction from the problematic work sustains those who respond to critical incidents. Vicarious posttraumatic growth occurs when listening to how others survive and thrive after traumatic events (Cohen & Collens, 2013). This growth results in resilience for both the trauma survivor and the first responder. Vicarious resilience counteracts the fatigue that could occur when trying to meet the needs of those who suffer (Ali et al., 2023). This vicarious resilience provides a profound strength that might not be present otherwise.

That is the benefit of providing care to those who suffer from trauma. The meaning-making process begins while forming new relationships. Everyone develops a new understanding of who they are and a greater appreciation for life (Barrington & Shakespeare-Finch, 2013). Providing trauma-informed care and practice for people is fulfilling. We hope that you follow your desire to help others. We can overcome the challenges we face in addressing trauma and helping those who have witnessed or experienced trauma. To do so requires becoming effective trauma workers and building communities of resilience.

A Flourishing Focus

Chapter Summary

Chapter 8 discusses the challenges in trauma work, including the assumptions about trauma work and the difficulties faced by professionals in providing help to traumatized clients. The chapter emphasizes the importance of ethical considerations in trauma work and the need for professionals to examine their motivations for working with trauma survivors. The chapter also discusses the ethical principles that guide trauma work, including autonomy, justice, beneficence, nonmaleficence, and fidelity.

The chapter highlights the systemic challenges in trauma work, such as the lack of clarity about terms used in the trauma field, the scarcity of research on measurements, and the neglect to care for clients with trauma. It also discusses the challenges faced by clients, including trauma disclosure avoidance, comorbid conditions, treatment adherence, and dropout. The chapter further explores clinicians' challenges, such as the lack of evidence-based training, clinician preference, and concerns about self-efficacy.

The chapter suggests potential solutions to these challenges, including cultivating knowledge and skills, promoting trauma-informed care, and developing resilience. It also emphasizes the importance of self-awareness and self-care for professionals working with trauma survivors.

Overall, the chapter highlights trauma work's complexity and unique nature and the need for professionals to approach it with sensitivity, ethical considerations, and a commitment to ongoing learning and growth.

Chapter Review

Please respond to the following questions:

1. What are the unique challenges trauma survivors face when seeking help and treatment?
2. What are the ethical considerations and challenges that therapists need to consider when working with trauma survivors?
3. How can organizations address the systemic challenges and barriers in trauma work?
4. What are the potential solutions and strategies to improve trauma-informed care and overcome the barriers clients and clinicians face?

Key Term Assessment

Review the following terms and try to explain each concept.

- Ethical principles
- Systemic challenges
- Therapy-interfering behaviors
- Boundaries
- Self-disclosure
- Self-efficacy

Resources

- The American Counseling Association has ethical guidelines for licensed professional counselors. The 2014 ACA Code of Ethics is available at: https://www.counseling.org/docs/default-source/ethics/2014-aca-code-of-ethics.pdf
- The American Psychological Association has published guidelines for education and training. A copy of the *Guidelines on Trauma Competencies for Education and Training* is available here: https://www.apa.org/ed/resources/trauma-competencies-training.pdf
- The Association of Traumatic Stress Specialists has a code of ethics for treating trauma.

The guidelines are available here: https://atss.info/wp-content/uploads/2022/04/code-of-ethics-04-15-2022.pdf

References

Ali, D. A., Figley, C. R., Tedeschi, R. G., Galarneau, D., & Amara, S. (2023). Shared trauma, resilience, and growth: A roadmap toward transcultural conceptualization. *Psychological Trauma: Theory, Research, Practice, and Policy, 15*(1), 45–55. https://doi.org/10.1037/tra0001044

Alpert, E., Gowdy-Jaehnig, A., Galovski, T. E., Meis, L. A., Polusny, M. A., Ackland, P. E., Spoont, M., Valenstein-Mah, H., Orazem, R. J., Schnurr, P. P., Chard, K. M., & Kehle-Forbes, S. M. (2024). Treatment-related beliefs and reactions among trauma-focused therapy completers and discontinuer: A qualitative examination. *Psychological Services.* Advance online publication. https://doi.org/10.1037/ser0000831

Anriani, H. B., Sari, H., Junaidi, J., & Hamka, H. (2022). Investigating the relationship between moral and ethical: Does extrinsic and intrinsic religiosity improve people's mental health? *FWU Journal of Social Science, 16*(3), 52–67. http://doi.org/10.51709/19951272/Fall2022/4

Aulia, K. N., Nadhirah, N. A., & Budiman, N. (2024). The dynamics of value imposition in counseling: Ethics and implications for the therapeutic relationship. *Student Scientific Creativity Journal, 2*(1). https://doi.org/10.55606/sscj-amik.v2i1.2674

Banaj, N., & Pellicano, C. (2020). Childhood trauma and stigma. In G. Spalletta, D. Janiri, F. Piras, & G. Sani (Eds.), *Childhood trauma in mental disorders*. Springer. https://doi.org/10.1007/978-3-030-49414-8_19

Barrington, A. J., & Shakespeare-Finch, J. (2013). Working with refugee survivors of torture and trauma: An opportunity for vicarious posttraumatic growth. *Counselling Psychology Quarterly, 26*(1), 89–105. https://doi.org/10.1080/09515070.2012.727553

Becker-Haimes, E. M., Wislocki, K., DiDonato, S., & Jensen-Doss, A. (2022). Predictors of clinician-reported self-efficacy in treating trauma-exposed youth. *Journal of Traumatic Stress, 35*(1), 109–119. https://doi.org/10.1002/jts.22688

Blundell, P., Oakley, L., & Kinmond, K. (2022). Who are we protecting? – Exploring counsellors' understanding and experience of boundaries. *European Journal for Qualitative Research in Psychotherapy, 12*, 13–28.

Brissett, D. I., Davies, S. H., & Sit, L. (2023). Reimagining no-shows as a symptom and not a diagnosis: A strength-based, trauma-sensitive approach. *Pediatrics, 151*(6), e2022057590. https://doi.org/10.1542/peds.2022-057590

Brown, L. S., & Courtois, C. A. (2019). Trauma treatment: The need for ongoing innovation. *Practice Innovations, 4*(3), 133–138. https://doi.org/10.1037/pri0000097

Brown, M. Z., & Dahlin, K. (2017). Dialectical behavior therapy for treating the effects of trauma. In S. N. Gold (Ed.), *APA handbook of trauma psychology: Volume 2 trauma practice* (pp. 275–294). American Psychological Association.

Carlisle, K. L., Levitt, D. H., & Neukrug, E. S. (2022). Mental health counselors' perceptions of ethical behaviors. *Counseling and Values, 67*(1), 88–115. https://doi.org/10.1163/2161007X-6701005

Carter, P., & Blanch, A. (2019). A trauma lens for systems change. *Stanford Social Innovation Review*, 47–54. https://www.napnappartners.org/sites/default/files/Trauma%20Lens%20for%20systems%20change_Stanford%20Social%20Innovation%20Review_2019.pdf

Champine, R. B., Lang, J. M., Nelson, A. M., Hanson, R. F., & Tebes, J. K. (2019). Systems measures of a trauma-informed approach: A systematic review. *American Journal of Community Psychology, 64*(3–4), 418–437. https://doi.org/10.1002/ajcp.12388

Cohen, K., & Collens, P. (2013). The impact of trauma work on trauma workers: A meta synthesis on vicarious trauma and vicarious posttraumatic growth. *Psychological Trauma: Theory, Research, Practice, and Policy, 5*(6), 570–580. https://doi.org/10.1037/a0030388

Coleman, A. M., Chouliara, Z., & Currie, K. (2018). Working in the field of complex psychological trauma: A framework for personal and professional growth, training, and supervision. *Journal of Interpersonal Violence, 36*(5–6), 2791–2815. https://doi.org/10.1177/0886260518759062

Cook, J. M., Newman, E., & Simiola, V. (2019). Trauma training: Competencies, initiatives, and resources. *Psychotherapy,* 56(3), 409–421. https://doi.org/10.1037/pst0000233

Cottone, R. R., Tarvydas, V. M., & Hartley, M. T. (2021). *Counseling ethics and decision making* (5th ed.). Springer Publishing Company.

De Boer, K., Arnold, C., Mackelprang, J. L., & Nedeljkovic, M. (2022). Barriers and facilitators to treatment seeking and engagement amongst women with complex trauma histories. *Health and Social Care in the Community.* https://doi.org/10.1111/hsc.13823

Delker, B. C., Salton, R., McLean, K. C., & Syed, M. (2020). Who has to tell their trauma story and how hard will it be? Influence of cultural stigma and narrative redemption on the storying of sexual violence. *PLoS One, 15*(6): e0234201. https://doi.org/10.1371/journal.pone.0234201

DeViva, J. C. (2014). Treatment utilization among OEF/OIF veterans referred for psychotherapy for PTSD. *Psychological Services, 11*(2), 179–184. https://doi.org/10.1037/a0035077

Espeleta, H. C., Peer, S. O., Are, F., & Hanson, R. F. (2022). Therapists' perceived competence in trauma-focused cognitive behavioral therapy and client outcomes: Findings from a community-based learning collaborative. *Child Maltreatment, 27*(3), 455–465. https://doi.org/10.1177/10775595211003673

Evaldas, K. (2017). Challenges for providing health care in traumatized populations: Barriers for PTSD treatments and the need for new developments, *Global Health Action, 10*(1). https://doi.org/10.1080/16549716.2017.1322399

Fernández, V., Gausereide-Corral, M., Valiente, C., & Sánchez-Iglesias, I. (2023). Effectiveness of trauma-informed care interventions at the organizational level: A systematic review. *Psychological Services, 20*(4), 849–863. https://doi.org/10.1037/ser0000737

Ferrell, E. L., Russin, S. E., & Grant, J. T. (2019). On being a client with posttraumatic stress disorder: Interactions with treatment providers and institutional barriers. *Journal of Community Psychology, 49*(3), 763–868. https://doi.org/10.1002/jcop.22359

Figley, C. R. (2002). Compassion fatigue: Psychotherapists' chronic lack of self care. *Journal of Clinical Psychology, 58*(11), 1433–1441. https://doi.org/10.1002/jclp.10090

Finch, J., Ford, C., Grainger, L., & Meiser-Stedman, R. (2020). A systematic review of the clinician related barriers and facilitators to the use of evidence-informed interventions for post traumatic stress. *Journal of Affective Disorders, 263,* 175–186. https://doi.org/10.1016/j.jad.2019.11.143

Finkstein, M., Stein, E., Greene, T., Bronstein, I., & Solomon, Z. (2015). Posttraumatic stress disorder and vicarious trauma in mental health professionals. *Health & Social Work, 40*(2), e25–e31. https://doi.org/10.1093/hsw/hlv026

Forester-Miller, H., & Davis, T. E. (2016). *Practitioner's guide to ethical decision making* (Rev. ed.). https://www.counseling.org/docs/default-source/ethics/practioner-39-s-guide-to-ethical-decision-making.pdf

Gjerstad, S. F., Nordin, L., Poulsen, S., Spadaro, E. F. A., & Palic, S. (2024). How is trauma-focused therapy experienced by adults with PTSD? A systematic review of qualitative studies. *BMC Psychology, 12*(1), 135. https://doi.org/10.1186/s40359-024-01588-x

Gnaulati, E. (2019). Potential ethical pitfalls and dilemmas in the promotion and use of American Psychological Association-recommended treatments for posttraumatic stress disorder. *Psychotherapy, 56*(3), 374–382. https://doi.org/10.1037/pst0000235

Gutheil, T., & Brodsky, A. (2008). *Preventing boundary violations in clinical practice.* Guilford Publications.

Holder, N., Holliday, R., Williams, R., Mullen, K., & Surís, A. (2018). A preliminary examination of the role of psychotherapist fidelity on outcomes of cognitive processing therapy during an RCT for military sexual trauma-related PTSD. *Cognitive Behaviour Therapy, 47*(1), 76–89. https://doi.org/10.1080/16506073.2017.1357750

Hoysted, C., Babl, F. E., Kassam-Adams, N., Landolt, M. A., Jobson, L., van der Westhuizen, C., Curtis, S., Kharbanda, A. B., Lyttle, M. D., Parri, N., Stanley, R., & Alisic, E. (2018). Knowledge and training in paediatric medical traumatic stress and trauma-informed care among emergency medical professionals in low- and middle-income countries. *European Journal of Psychotraumatology, 9*(1), Article 1468703. https://doi.org/10.1080/2000819 8.2018.1468703

Jenks, D. B., & Oka, M. (2022). Breaking hearts: Ethically handling transference and counter-transference in therapy. *The American Journal of Family Therapy, 49*(5), 443–460. https://doi.org/10.1080/01926187.2020.1830732

Johnson, M. K., Weeks, S. N., Peacock, G. G., & Domenech Rodríguez, M. M. (2022). Ethical decision-making models: A taxonomy of models and review of issues. *Ethics & Behavior, 32*(3), 195–209. https://doi.org/10.1080/10508422.2021.113593

Jolley, H. K. (2019). I'm human too: Person-centred counsellors' lived experiences of therapist self-disclosure. *European Journal of Qualitative Research in Psychotherapy, 9*, 12–26. http://ejqrp.org/index.php/ejqrp/article/view/54

Kantor, V., Knefel, M., & Lueger-Schuster, B. (2017). Perceived barriers and facilitators of mental health service utilization in adult trauma survivors: A systematic review. *Clinical Psychology Review, 52*, 52–68. https://doi.org/10.1016/j.cpr.2016.12.001

Kazlauskas, E. (2017). Challenges for providing health care in traumatized populations: Barriers for PTSD treatments and the need for new developments. *Global Health Action, 10*(1), 1322399. https://doi.org/10.1080/16549716.2017.1322399

Kehle-Forbes, S., Meis, L. A., Spoont, M. R., & Polusny, M. A. (2016). Treatment initiation and dropout from prolonged exposure and cognitive processing therapy in a VA outpatient clinic.

Psychological Trauma: Theory, Research, Practice, and Policy, 8(1), 107–114. https://doi.org/10.1037/tra0000065

Kehle-Forbes, S. M., Ackland, P. E., Spoont, M. R., Meis, L. A., Orazem, R. J., Lyon, A., Valentein-Mah, H. R., Schnurr, P. P., Zickmund, S. L., Foa, E. B., Chard, K. M., Alpert, E., & Polusny, M. A. (2022). Divergent experience of U.S. veterans who did and did not complete trauma-focused therapies for PTSD: A national qualitative study of treatment dropout. *Behaviour Research and Therapy, 154*, Article 104123. https://doi.org/10.1016/j.brat.2022.104123

Kerns, S. E. U., Cevasco, M., Comtois, K. A., Dorsey, S., King, K., McMahon, R., Sedlar, G., Lee, T. G., Mazza, J. J., Lengua, L., Davis, C., Evans-Campbell, T., Trupin, E. W. (2016). An interdisciplinary university-based initiative for graduate training in evidence-based treatments for children's mental health. *Journal of Emotional & Behavioral Disorders, 24*(1), 3–15. https://doi.org/10.1177/1063426615583457

Kim, J. J., Brookman-Frazee, L., Gellatly, R., Stadnick, N., Barnett, M. L., & Lau, A. S. (2018). Predictors of burnout among community therapists in the sustainment phase of a system-driven implementation of multiple evidence-based practices in children's mental health. *Professional Psychology: Research and Practice, 49*(2), 132–141. https://doi.org/10.1037/pro0000182

Kirst, M., Aery, A., Matheson, F. I., & Stergiopoulos, V. (2017). Provider and consumer perceptions of trauma-informed practices and services for substance use and mental health problems. *International Journal of Mental Health and Addiction, 15*, 514–528. https://doi.org/10.1007/s11469-016-9693-z

Kitchener, K. S. (1984). Intuition, critical evaluation, and ethical principles: The foundation for ethical decisions in counseling psychology. *The Counseling Psychologist, 12*(3), 43–55. https://doi.org/10.1177/0011000084123005

Kitchener, K. S., & Anderson, S. K. (2011). *Foundations of ethical practice, research, and teaching in psychology and counseling* (2nd ed.). Routledge.

Knight, C. (2019). Trauma-informed practice and care: Implications for field instruction. *Clinical Social Work Journal, 47*, 79–89. https://doi.org/10.1007/s10615-018-0661-x

Konya, J., Perôt, C., Pitt, K., Johnson, E., Gregory, A., Brown, E., Feder, G., & Campbell, J. (2020). Peer-led groups for survivors of sexual abuse and assault: A systematic review. *Journal of Mental Health*, 1–13. https://doi.org/10.1080/09638237.2020.1770206

Lambert, M. J., Hansen, N. B., & Finch, A. E. (2001). Patient-focused research: Using patient outcome data to enhance treatment effects. *Journal of Consulting and Clinical Psychology, 69*, 159–172. https://doi.org/10.1037/0022-006X.69.2.159

Lashkay, A.-M., Kinsella, E. L., & Muldoon, O. T. (2023). When trauma is stigmatized: Disidentification and dissociation in people affected by adverse childhood experiences. *Journal of Community & Applied Social Psychology, 33*(5), 1225–1240. https://doi.org/10.1002/casp.2702

Leung, T., Schmidt, F., & Mushquash, C. (2023). A personal history of trauma and experience of secondary traumatic stress, vicarious trauma, and burnout in mental health workers: A systematic literature review. *Psychological Trauma: Theory, Research, Practice, and Policy, 15*(Suppl 2), S213–S221. https://doi.org/10.1037/tra0001277

Levenson, J. (2017). Trauma-informed social work practice. *Social Work, 62*(2), 105–113. https://doi.org/10.1093/sw/swx001

Lin, Y.-K., Liu, K.-T., Chen, C.-W., Lee, W.-C., Lin, C.-J., Shi, L., & Tien, Y.-C. (2019). How to effectively obtain informed consent in trauma patients: A systematic review. *BMC Medical Ethics, 20*(1), 8. https://doi.org/10.1186/s12910-019-0347-0

LoParo, D., Florez, I. A., Valentine, N., & Lamis, D. A. (2019). Associations of suicide prevention trainings with practices and confidence among clinicians at community mental health centers. *Suicide and Life-Threatening Behavior, 49*(4), 1148–1156. https://doi.org/10.1111/sltb.12498

Marques, L., Dixon, L., Valentine, S. E., Borba, C. P. C., Simon, N. M., & Wiltsey Stirman, S. (2016). Providers' perspectives of factors influencing implementation of evidence-based treatments in a community mental health setting: A qualitative investigation of the training–practice gap. *Psychological Services, 13*(3), 322–331. https://doi.org/10.1037/ser0000087

May, J. M., Richardi, T. M., & Barth, K. S. (2016). Dialectical behavior therapy as treatment for borderline personality disorder. *Mental Health Clinician, 6*(2), 62–67. https://doi.org/10.9740/mhc.2016.03.62

McElvaney, R. (2015). Disclosure of child sexual abuse: Delays, non-disclosure and partial disclosure. What the research tells us and implications for practice. *Child Abuse Review, 24*(3), 159–169. https://doi.org/10.1002/car.2280

Melaki, E., & Stavrou, P.-D. (2023). Re-exploring the vicarious posttraumatic growth and trauma: A comparison study between private therapists and therapists in nonprofit organizations treating trauma survivors. *Traumatology, 29*(1), 27–35. https://doi.org/10.1037/trm0000378

Menschner, C. & Maul, A. (2016, April). *Key Ingredients for successful trauma-informed care implementation.* Substance Abuse and Mental Health Services Administration. https://www.samhsa.gov/sites/default/files/programs_campaigns/childrens_mental_health/atc-whitepaper-040616.pdf

Mott, J. M., Mondragon, S., Hundt, N. E., Beason-Smith, M., Grady, R. H., & Teng, E. J. (2014). Characteristics of U.S. veterans who begin and complete prolonged exposure and cognitive processing therapy for PTSD. *Journal of Traumatic Stress, 27*(3), 265–273. https://doi.org/10.1002/jts.21927

Mueller, J., Moergeli, H., & Maercker, A. (2008). Disclosure and social acknowledgement as predictors of recovery from posttraumatic stress: A longitudinal study in crime victims. *Canadian Journal of Psychiatry, 53*(3), 160–168. https://doi.org/10.1177/070674370805300306

Oramas, J. E. (2017). Counseling ethics: Overview of challenges, responsibilities and recommended practices. *Journal of Multidisciplinary Research, 9*(3), 47–58.

Quinn, D. M., Williams, M. K., Quintana, F., Gaskins, J. L., Overstreet, N. M., Pishori, A., Earnshaw, V. A., Perez, G., & Chaudoir, S. R. (2014). Examining effects of anticipated stigma, centrality, salience, internalization, and outness on psychological distress for people with concealable stigmatized identities. *PLoS One, 9*(5), e96977. https://doi.org/10.1371/journal.pone.0096977

Rizvi, S. F. B., Batool, S. F., & Sajid, U. (2021). Ethical aspects when treating traumatized subjects. *Pakistan Journal of Ethics, 1*(1), 3–8.

Robotham, D., Sweeney, A., & Perôt, C. (2019). Violence, abuse and mental health network: Survivors' priority themes and questions for research — Consultation report, 2019. https://www.vamhn.co.uk/uploads/1/2/2/7/122741688/consultation_report_on_website.pdf

Salyers, M. P., Evans, L. J., Bond, G. R., & Meyer, P. S. (2004). Barriers to assessment and treatment of posttraumatic stress disorder and other trauma-related problems in people with severe mental illness: Clinician perspectives. *Community Mental Health Journal, 40*, 17–31. https://doi.org/10.1023/B:COMH.0000015215.45696.5f

Shapiro, C. J., MacDonell, K. W., & Moran, M. (2021). Provider self-efficacy in delivering evidence-based psychosocial interventions: A scoping review. *Implementation Research and Practice, 2*. https://doi.org/10.1177/2633489520988258

Siddique, J. (2018). Toward a new paradigm of health and human potential. *World Futures, 74*(2), 116–133. https://doi.org/10.1080/02604027.2018.1427334

Sijercic, I., Liebman, R. E., Stirman, S. W., & Monson, C. M. (2021). The effect of therapeutic alliance on dropout in cognitive processing therapy for posttraumatic stress disorder. *Journal of Traumatic Stress, 34*, 819–828. https://doi.org/10.1002/jts.22676

Sire, J. (2020). *The universe next door: A basic worldview catalog.* IVP Academic.

Skar, A. M. S., Braathu, N., Jensen, T. K., & Ormhaug, S. M. (2022). Predictors of nonresponse and dropout among children and adolescents receiving TF-CBT: Investigation of client-, therapist-, and implementation factors. *BMC Health Services Research, 22*, Article 1212. https://doi.org/10.1186/s12913-022-08497-y

Stamm, B. H. (1995). Professional quality of life scale (PROQOL) [Database record]. *APA PsycTests.* https://doi.org/10.1037/t05192-000

Stark, C., Tapia-Fuselier, J. L., Jr., & Bunch, K. (2022). The trauma-informed ethical decision-making model: An integrative framework. *Journal of Trauma Studies in Education, 1*(1), 86–103. https://doi.org/10.32674/jis.v1i1.3678

Tener, D., & Murphy, S. B. (2015). Adult disclosure of child sexual abuse: A literature review. *Trauma, Violence, & Abuse, 16*(4), 391–400. https://doi.org/10.1177/1524838014537906

Trottier, K., Monson, C. M., Wonderlich, S. A., MacDonald, D. E., & Olmsted, M. P. (2017). Frontline clinicians' perspectives on and utilization of trauma-focused therapy with individuals with eating disorders. *Eating Disorders, 1*, 22–36. https://doi.org/10.1080/10640266.2016.1207456

References

U.S. Government Accountability Office (GAO). (2024, March 5). The mismatch between mental health care access and demand. https://www.gao.gov/blog/mismatch-between-mental-health-care-access-and-demand

Unjai, S., Forster, E. M., Mitchell, A. E., & Creedy, D. K. (2022). Compassion satisfaction, resilience and passion for work among nurses and physicians working in intensive care units: A mixed method systematic review. *Intensive & Critical Care Nursing, 71*, 103248. https://doi.org/10.1016/j.iccn.2022.103248

Wagner, B., Keller, V., Knaevelsrud, C., & Maercker, A. (2012). Social acknowledgement as a predictor of posttraumatic stress and complicated grief after witnessing assisted suicide. *International Journal of Social Psychiatry, 58*(4), 381–385. https://doi.org/10.1177/0020764011400791

Wathen, C. N., Schmitt, B., & MacGregor, J. C. D. (2023). Measuring trauma- (and violence-) informed care: A scoping review. *Trauma, Violence, & Abuse, 24*(1), 261–277. https://doi.org/10.1177/15248380211029399

Welfel, E. R. (2016). *Ethics in counseling & psychotherapy* (6th ed.). Cengage Learning.

Yang, S., Schneider, B., Wynn, G. H., & Howe, E., III. (2017). Ethical considerations in the treatment of PTSD in military populations. *Focus: The Journal of Lifelong Learning in Psychiatry, 15*(4), 435–440. https://doi.org/10.1176/appi.focus.20170035

Chapter Nine
Becoming Effective Providers in Resilient Communities

Overview
Effective Trauma Workers
Developing Trauma Competency
Creating a Trauma-Sensitive World
A Flourishing Focus
Chapter Summary
References

Overview

Chapter 9: Becoming Effective Providers in Resilient Communities explores the characteristics of effective trauma workers, emphasizing the necessity of self-awareness, emotion regulation, and the ability to build and maintain therapeutic relationships. It emphasizes the need for competency training among professionals across various fields to enhance trauma care skills. The chapter discusses the challenges faced by individuals with trauma in healthcare, education, and legal systems, highlighting the need for trauma-informed approaches to prevent mismanagement of situations. Chapter 9 underscores the importance of developing trauma-informed communities and outlines the process, from engaging advocates to educating community members and implementing new policies and approaches. Stressing the necessity of transforming community perspectives occurs as this chapter offers practices to become trauma-informed and develop systems of care. The chapter concludes with a discussion of the creation of resilient societies, stressing the importance of collective strength, joint capacities, and the need for interaction and cooperation.

Effective Trauma Workers

We have watched various people work with trauma survivors through the years and are amazed at who is most effective at this work. Some people have natural skills in relating to others, and some do not have the relational basics. Some people have

DOI: 10.4324/9781003463009-9

the training and yet are not relatable. Therefore, it is essential to discuss the characteristics of effective trauma workers, which include deepening our self and other awareness, sustaining a non-anxious presence, building and maintaining therapeutic relationships, and developing competency (Baranowsky, 2019; Miller & Sprang, 2017).

Maintaining Self and Other Awareness

First, those who work in trauma must have self-awareness of how they interact with others. In a previous chapter, we discussed a question that is essential in supporting others. "Whose need does this meet?" This reflection is important as we work with trauma survivors. Often, we have a desire to help. While altruistic, it also meets a deep need within some to find meaning and significance in this world. Yet, sometimes our efforts to assist end up benefiting us more than the person we are trying to help. While you may not like a manualized approach to trauma, the value of such is that it serves as a manager for the countertransference we experience as people who care. We would be foolish if we did not acknowledge that working with others makes us feel good or gives us the opportunity to work on our own psychological or relational issues. That desire is not immoral but may not be in the client's best interest. Therefore, we recommend therapists engage in personal therapy. Steve describes their observation of this in a well-meaning but misdirected partner.

> I observed a therapy dog owner talking to the victims about a prior incident involving children just weeks before. I pulled him aside and queried him about his intention. It seemed he wanted to let everyone know his dog served in that incident, but I reminded him to stay in the present moment with these people who needed to process their trauma. Besides that, his role as a silent witness and let the dog do the work. Telling stories of his accomplishments was not his role. His lack of self-awareness was frustrating and had the potential to harm those who had traumatic stress symptoms. This dog owner may have been unaware that we were in a medical office where physicians involved in the incident were moved just days after the shooting episode.

While we want to respect this man for the service he offers and note that this gives him pleasure to do so, we must also remind ourselves that what we do for others is best attained in our present accompaniment in their journey. Sometimes in therapy, we prioritize our own pleasure over the client's needs. Being a crisis counselor requires high self-awareness and calmness (Ray et al., 2013). That is what Steve was trying to do on that day while they walked the hallways of the medical office. Maintaining a present awareness of our thoughts, emotions, and motivations during the counseling helps us to maintain a healthy detachment. That also protects us from burnout and secondary trauma (Ludick & Figley, 2017; Van der Merwe & Hunt, 2019).

Active self and other awareness occur when the effective trauma worker notices the surrounding environment and the potential for re-traumatization. They commit to providing physical and psychological safety for people (Pohl et al., 2021). In another conversation, a higher education professional explained their reaction during the Hurricane Katrina crisis. As news poured in via the television station, she told her senior administrator, "We should change the station to a different channel. This constant news could become traumatizing if this is the only station option available in the student union building." Her concern was for those students who already had trauma and how watching further traumatic news could increase their PTSD symptoms. An effective trauma worker normalizes the trauma reactions of people and commits to providing physical and psychological safety for people (Pohl et al., 2021).

Sustaining a Non-Anxious Presence

Other characteristics include the ability to regulate emotional responses during clients' intense affective and behavioral dysregulation (Bosk et al., 2020). When the trauma worker manages their physiological reactivity, it protects them from secondary trauma while providing co-regulation for the client (Gentry et al., 2017; Miller & Sprang, 2017). This practice of self-regulation serves as a model to clients in teaching them how to modulate uncomfortable tension in stressful situations with an activated sympathetic nervous system (Gentry et al., 2017). In this way, the trauma worker is showing the individual how to manage their stress in the present moment while maintaining a healthy relationship. This can occur when therapists teach clients how to take deep, calming breaths, or how to shift from a hypervigilant state to a peaceful one. Some activities to accomplish this may include progressive muscle relaxation or showing a client how to tense and relax muscle groups. We caution helpers against using the word, relax, as it triggers the opposite response. Instead, use "tighten and let go" or "tense and release". Another useful self-regulation skill that can be used is to have the individual say to themself, "Soften. Soften your face. Soften your body." This works well when surrounded by people and can create calmness. We want clients to attune to the feelings and thoughts that accompany the physical sensation so they can learn to adapt and use these skills throughout the day.

Building Relationships

Healing for trauma occurs in a healthy relationship. That is why the helper must resolve their primary trauma and attachment issues. People who experience childhood trauma may have insecure attachments, often repeated in relational patterns that further exacerbate their traumatic stress (Bosk et al., 2020). Traumatized individuals might have difficulty with trust and, therefore, have trouble establishing relationships that bring healing. Instead, they develop a negative schema wherein they tell themselves they do not deserve love, affection, or attention. This shame blocks their ability to process their trauma and reduces their motivation, leading to hopelessness and helplessness (Melegkovits et al., 2023). They need unconditional support from a trustworthy person who can witness their narrative as a gentle witness. However, gaining that initial trust requires patience. It takes time.

Belinda, a licensed therapist, describes her work with trauma in the following way.

> I remember meeting Alice when she was 19. She requested help after enduring abandonment by her biological mother and father, molestation at 14 by her adoptive father, and ongoing abuse by her adoptive mother. She was an overachiever and arrived in the office at the request of her pastor. Alice was a beautiful young woman but feared abandonment. As a result, she pursued men who were unavailable or uninterested and then experience repeated rejection. Alice was consuming alcohol during the week. I confronted her about her behaviors, and she was shocked that I did, but it captured her attention. It took about six months before she trusted me, but all the pain she had experienced poured out once she did. Once she trusted, we could begin the hard work. Before that, her behavior was erratic, and her therapy attendance was sporadic. My job was to be patient and full of grace with her. I knew she was trying her best and needed time to believe that I would be around for her.

A different clinician, Russell, explained how he built a relationship with a client who had complex traumatic events that interfered with her life.

> Sally taught me how to be a trauma counselor. She had been hospitalized sixteen times within four years when I first met her, molested by her father, assaulted in her early 20s, experienced domestic violence with her spouse in her 30s, and entered therapy with me while she had three young children. She was suicidal weekly, which interfered with treatment progress. It took two years and two hospitalizations for her to trust. Finally, she learned I had

her best interests at heart, and she took some forward steps. Over the next year, she learned how to manage her suicidality and practice emotion regulation. I learned how to move slowly, how to pace treatment, and how to help her best when and where she needed it. We built and maintained the type of relationship that she needed during that time. What I needed was further training to develop trauma competency.

These two examples show how, with patience and time, the clients trusted their therapists and made progress. Both clinicians offered a safe place for their clients. There are times when a professional feel they are not doing enough. These stories reveal that just providing a caring and non-anxious presence can be therapeutic.

Nurture Understanding

Consider the following case. Jason shared his dismay at the loss of his primary care physician, who retired and whose office had recently closed. The office staff were trained in trauma-informed care. Jason has PTSD and so showing up for his appointments was difficult until he found this physician. He regularly attended his appointments with the physician assistant. The receptionist was friendly and kind. There was never a long office wait, and when called back to the exam room, the medical assistant would ask him about his fishing hobby first. Then she would proceed with obtaining his vitals and basic information. The physician assistant would address his concerns and then set aside her laptop. Looking at him, she would probe gently, "Jason, how are you really doing today?" He knew she cared. This wasn't therapy, but just that she asked made him feel connected to his healthcare team. Jason was reassigned to a physician at another clinic. He waited two months to see him. The receptionist was not unfriendly. She asked for the requisite information, but never looked at Jason. The medical assistant gathered Jason's vitals without offering him reassurance or informing him of the results. The doctor entered the room and immediately informed him he had resigned and would not be his doctor after the month ended. Then the physician gave his rationale. Jason, who had difficulty trusting anyway, felt abandoned by the system. He had been re-traumatized, albeit unintentionally, by a new office that was not trauma-informed. Now it will be difficult for Jason to continue his medications and follow up with his medical care:

- How could the new medical office become trauma-informed?
- In what way could their practices change that is simple to implement?
- What suggestions do you have for Jason?

Developing Trauma Competency

Different ways exist in which one builds competency in trauma-informed care. One can do so in the following ways: on-the-job experience, peer learning, through seminars, workshops, or other online or in-person workshops, or through a certification program. Multiple paths exist, and each person must determine how they can learn best. The Substance Abuse and Mental Health Services Administration offers trauma training for criminal justice professionals through the GAINS Center for Behavioral Health and Justice Transformation (SAMHSA, 2024). Many courses are available for medical providers, educators, and legal advocates in trauma-informed care. Counselors can obtain training through continuing education in much the same way.

Unfortunately, graduate counseling programs offer few trauma courses to develop the needed competencies for students. In a study of 193 APA-accredited programs, only 5% required a course in trauma-informed care. This means only 8% of graduating doctoral students had a single course in trauma (Foltz et al., 2023; Henning et al., 2022). Training programs accredited by the Council for Accreditation of Counseling and Related Education Programs (CACREP), considered the gold standard for graduate counseling programs offer little trauma-informed training with only 3.4% of the programs offering a stand-alone course in trauma-informed care (Mathew et al., 2023). We suggest that graduate programs and licensing boards require more than one trauma course for emerging professionals. Scientific knowledge, an overview of trauma, and practice skills produce confidence in the person who desires to work with traumatized individuals. Without knowledge or practice, it is difficult to develop competency (Taylor, 2016).

The lack of training among professionals, including mental health providers, is troublesome and may harm trauma survivors. Without proper education, a person may not recognize trauma, provide an inaccurate diagnosis, or mistreat clients because of inaccurate assessments and inadequate treatment plans (Cook & Newman, 2017). In a survey of 1,946 psychiatric patients who screened positive for PTSD, almost 14% were undetected by their clinicians (Lewis et al., 2018). Not only are there challenges in trauma-informed practice, but there are also potential risks for those who provide such care.

Because of the lack of trauma competency training, a consortium gathered to discuss the remedies to this problem. In April 2013, Yale University sponsored a national conference entitled "Advancing the Science of Education, Training and Practice in Trauma" to identify competencies for trauma. These included the foundational and functional skills necessary for knowledge and treatment that were necessary components (Cook et al., 2019). Eight competencies, called the New Haven Competencies, were approved by the American Psychological Association (APA) as the official guidelines for education and training in the United States (APA, 2015).

These guidelines specify five categories of competencies: scientific knowledge about trauma, psychosocial trauma-focused assessment, trauma-focused psychosocial intervention, trauma-informed professionalism, and trauma-informed relational and systems. The scientific knowledge about trauma refers to one's ability to recognize, respect, evaluate, and apply the knowledge in appropriate and ethical ways. Assessment means applying current assessments measures that are normed, validated, and psychometrically suitable for use with traumatized clients (Cook et al., 2014). Interventions should be evidence-based and include pharmacological and psychological treatments that emphasize a client's strengths, and prioritize openness, safety, and trust, while decreasing avoidance. The interventions should also seek to facilitate effective collaboration with families, groups, and systems. Professionalism includes the values, skills, and attitudes that include working ethically on behalf of trauma survivors, and in relationships and systems (Cook & Newman, 2017; Cook et al., 2014). The components are necessary for the assessment and care for the training, research, assessment, and care of individuals with trauma and set the minimum standard necessary for trauma workers who desire to work in the field (Figure 9.1).

While these guidelines exist, there appears to be minor oversight to ensure these competencies are present in counselors in the field. Given the immense workload of state boards responsible for licensing counselors, there is minimal opportunity to evaluate a therapist's ability to provide trauma care competently. While state regulations may prohibit licensed providers from claiming to be experts in areas in which they do not have additional or specialized training, the lack of oversight does not prevent therapists from claiming expertise. They may be, indeed, helpful to many

Developing Trauma Competency

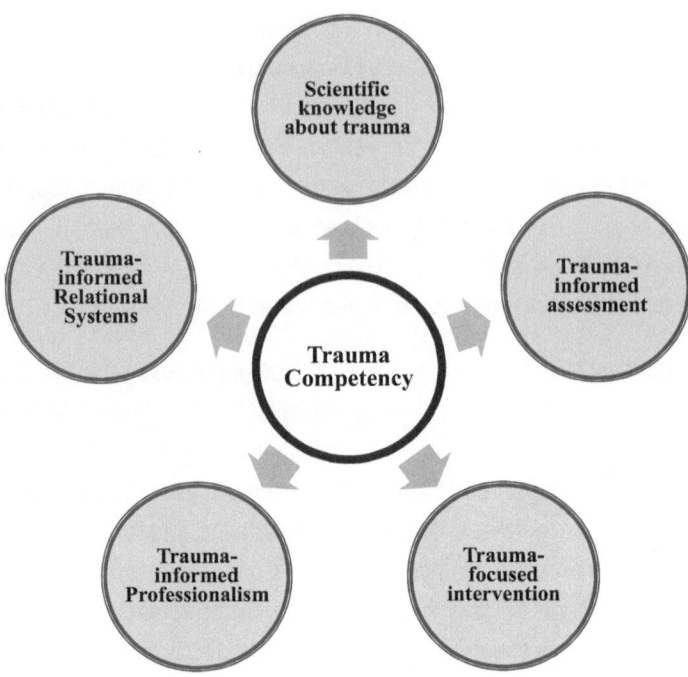

FIGURE 9.1 Trauma Competencies.

(Cook & Newman, 2017).

people, but they could also be harmful to clients. At present, the best we can do is encourage them to obtain the needed education and training to treat trauma survivors.

Creating a Trauma-Sensitive World

When adopting a new worldview, one must begin with basic assumptions. This means asking questions about how things exist and what causes them to happen. It also means developing hypotheses about solutions for problems. To create a trauma-sensitive world, we must ask the following questions:

- Does trauma exist? How prevalent is it in my community? Does it affect a few, some, or many people in the community?
- How do we know trauma exists? What are the signs and symptoms of trauma in individuals, families, groups, and our community? How long have these signs been present?

- How should we use the knowledge we have learned to help individuals, families, groups, and our community?
- What changes do we need to make to integrate trauma-informed care into system policies, procedures, and practices? In what ways can we seek to actively resist re-traumatizing individuals, families, groups, or our community?

(SAMHSA, 2014)

Specific services areas or types of professionals may alter the implementation. It means that from the moment a person or family contact the agency or enter the community, all staff members, including receptionists, intake employees, direct care personnel, managers, supervisors, administrators, law enforcement, educators, legal advocates, board members, clergy, and hospitality personnel understand how to provide trauma-informed care to all people (SAMHSA, 2014). This requires a deep commitment to building competency through recruitment, hiring practices, retention, and training. It means forming collaborative service systems to provide continuity of care throughout the community. In addition, a trauma-focused view requires a community to embed the following principles into systems of care: safety, trust, collaboration, choice, empowerment, and sensitivity to cultural, historical, and gender issues (Knight, 2018).

The process of developing a trauma-sensitive community involves engaging counselors, educators, judges, and other community leaders to be advocates who offer to speak on behalf of creating such a system. These promoters should use a common language with the universal understanding, empowering everyone they encounter to create organizational and community cultural change. The process includes educating everyone in trauma-informed care and working in collaboration to provide continuity of care. The system should include evaluation strategies to ensure effectiveness and addresses barriers or challenges that arise (Clements et al., 2020). It can also offer practical guidelines for providers throughout the system, including medical providers, first responders, educators, legal advocates, clergy, and counselors.

Building trauma-informed communities requires not only a paradigm shift, but also action steps. The community will need to identify and form partnerships. This can occur by offering education about trauma and systems of care to those working in

Creating a Trauma-Sensitive World

healthcare, emergency services, law enforcement, education, legal services, religious settings, and other organizations who interact with the public (Haas & Clements, 2019). As this occurs, community members develop further awareness of and sensitivity to trauma and adopt new policies and approaches in their work.

Medical Providers

Educating medical providers incorporates an understanding of the overloaded systems in which these professionals operate, the pressures they face, and ensuring that becoming trauma-informed will be beneficial. It is important that healthcare workers realize moving to trauma-informed care lessens their stress load rather than increasing their duties or demands. When the medical system operates with a trauma-informed perspective and adopts recommended approaches, they increase their individual compassion satisfaction, and therefore decrease the risk of burnout (Elisseou et al., 2024). The medical system communicates better with patients, external constituents, and internal operations, increasing patient satisfaction and cooperation. Implementing this trauma focus increases screening and provides aid more quickly, resulting in reduced depression and anxiety, increased patient acknowledgement of traumatic events, and improved mental and physical health (Chin et al., 2024).

The previous story about Jason illustrates how a lack of trauma education might impact a patient negatively and possibly re-traumatize them. A few simple practices at the new office could have changed the outcome. Once the physician resigned, the office could have contacted Jason and provided him with an opportunity to choose a different physician ahead of time. Upon arrival, a simple smile and saying, "Welcome. We're so glad you're here," would help ease Jason's fear of being in a new office. The medical assistant could let Jason know his weight, his blood pressure, and any other vitals she took, as well as approximately how long until the doctor might arrive. These practices would only take a few seconds. Often, people assume that providing trauma-informed care disrupts a busy system when it only requires a sensitivity and understanding of human nature.

Providing trauma-informed care means showing compassion toward patients. A recent development in traumatology is the science of compassionomics, the study of how compassionate care affects patient health, providers, and the healthcare system. Research into primary care and hospital settings reveals that healthcare providers miss opportunities for compassionate response in around 70% of their patient encounters. Unfortunately, the studies also show that a clinician interrupts a patient after 11 seconds, thus indicating a lack of understanding of trauma-informed care (Levinson et al., 2000; Weiss et al., 2017). In his research, Trzeciak states that 40 seconds of active listening increases patient satisfaction and reduces provider burnout (Trzeciak & Mazzarelli, 2019). Recommendations for creating trauma-informed organization change suggested by Elisseou et al. (2024) include incorporating a trauma-informed approach in the organization's core mission, communicating in respectful and transparent ways, and increasing collaboration with patients and key concerned individuals. These initial steps can lead the way to enhancing everyone's experience in health care services.

First Responders

The difficulty for emergency responders is prioritizing the need. For firefighters, emergency medical service personnel, or law enforcement, there is an acute need to attend to the urgent situation quickly and responsibly. It makes sense and we do not want to slow this process. However, understanding trauma should facilitate in speeding up and ensuring participant responses. Trauma is a sensory experience. For a person with a history of trauma, or for a person experiencing a trauma, they will be in a heightened sense of arousal, emotion dysregulation, sensory sensitivity, avoidance, and may dissociate. These complicate engagement with the traumatized person.

Law enforcement officers frequently interact with people who have mental health conditions, including schizophrenia, substance-related disorders, affective disorders, and PTSD. Unfortunately, stigmatization of individuals with a mental health diagnosis is common, and those interacting with them may believe they are dangerous if their behavior appears erratic. Along with the increase in pressure and dysregulation that an officer may experience in such encounters, misfortunate altercations may occur, resulting in injury or arrest (Lorey & Fegert, 2022). Training for law enforcement and emergency responders may be helpful in producing more positive outcomes. Collaboration within systems of care can provide the additional support needed for traumatized individuals and first responders.

Key strategies for emergency responders will be to use their own calmness to co-regulate or bring a sense of calmness in the person experiencing the trauma. Being gentle, kind, and reassuring even though firm will help. Explain what is happening,

Creating a Trauma-Sensitive World

what you are doing, and why you are doing it. If possible, provide a private setting, acknowledge the person's bravery, and ask how they are feeling. Using a trauma-informed approach can improve the quality of the person's response, the report they give, and how they cooperate (Rich, 2019; Wexler, 2024). The advantage you have is the unique position in providing clear information about the situation, safety plans, and access to trauma-informed professional services or peer support.

Educators

Teachers can incorporate trauma-informed practices in the classroom. They have such an arduous task of managing a group of children throughout the day, all with varying needs. One useful model to help is the Tri-Phasic Model, which highlights three basic needs for children: safety and stabilization, remembrance, and mourning, and re-engagement (Morton, 2022). When a child or teen needs safety and stabilization, they have a prime need for connection. Typically, their behaviors will be attention-seeking. Although punishing poor behavior may appear logical, it is important to remember that negative punishment does not effectively alter such behaviors. In fact, punish-ment reinforces negative behaviors. During these times, children need attunement, emotional, and physical safety. They need to be seen and valued (Morton, 2022). This might be a time to assign them a task where they can be successful or receive an award or be a helper. It may be a time for a breathing or stretching exercise.

One day Jeannie came and said that Johnny should not come back to the after-school program at church. The director, Sam, requested the reason. Jeannie explained Johnny was misbehaving and distracting the other children. Sam said, "Jeannie, did it occur to you that Johnny needs some attention? His parents are drug users, and his grandpa doesn't really take care of him. If we don't let him come, then who's going to take care of him? Why don't you give Johnny a way to help you?" Reluctantly, Jeannie went back to her class. She tried what Sam suggested. While Johnny continued to struggle, he settled. Best of all, Jeannie realized that maybe the message that this group cared about Johnny might help him survive the rest of life.

The second part of the Tri-Phasic Model is remembrance and mourning. When a child or adolescent experiences trauma, they may have times when they are in pain or experience triggers. They may become hypervigilant, angry, or emotional. At these times, they need coaching, stabilization, and emotion regulation (Morton, 2022). This is an ideal time for the teacher to show mindfulness skills, deep breathing, use music, or rhythmic activities. Or if the child is struggling to be still or remain seated, then a teacher can provide sensory supports, like a fidget item, weighted lap pad, noise-cancelling headphones, or kinetic sand. They can also provide a calming corner (Norrish & Brunzell, 2023).

During the third phase, re-engagement, the child, or adolescent, needs the opportunity to use their brain and build their emotional skills (Morton, 2022). This is when they can think about what just happened and identify a different action choice for the next time. Unfortunately, this is where most teachers start, but children cannot begin here until the first two phases are completed. Implementing this plan will be more rewarding for educators and students alike.

Legal Advocates

For legal advocates, many of the same principles apply. Albrink (2023) clarifies that you do not shift from being an attorney to a therapist. That is not what being trauma-informed implies. Instead, it means that you enhance your services to clients through your cognizance of their physical, emotional, psychological, sociological, and physiological needs. Having a trauma-informed perspective informs how you communicate, litigate, represent, and interact with your client, and do so in a way that does not re-traumatize your client. Albrink (2023) makes several suggestions for legal practice. These include offering a welcoming and safe environment that is accessible, being sensitive and aware of systemic racism and historical trauma and providing resources that meet a variety of client needs. Albrink (2023) also recommends that legal advocates examine the firm's transparency and provide clarity to clients when needed. Legal staff and employees can be trained in trauma sensitivity and implicit bias to prevent unintentional harm (Albrink, 2023). These practices are simple and will provide your clients with the best services while promoting good will throughout the community.

Clergy

Trauma is not a mystery to the church. Whether a person attends a synagogue, mosque, tabernacle, or other structure, or even if they are not a member of a religious organization, they often seek help from a religious leader during difficult times. The church, or community of believers, is in a unique position to respond with care. Regrettably,

Creating a Trauma-Sensitive World

there are instances when that cannot occur. Clergy must ensure that they and their congregants or followers receive training in trauma-informed practices. They can accept the person with trauma without adding shame, to accommodate this person who may have difficulty trusting, or following through with commitments. The church can practice being non-judgmental and be the place for struggle and doubt. Providing a safe and comfortable place that allows choices, instead of exertion of power and control. The church can provide safeguarding policies that protect everyone (Singer, 2024). The leader, or clergy, can use delicate words to encourage attenders to become their best selves, instead of condemning them or highlighting their failures. Moving from a shame-based model to a celebration of new life and hope that change can happen is a trauma-informed approach. Clergy can offer to support people amid their struggles, not asking them to leave when they do not fit in. These are the practices that encourage people to grow and heal.

Whenever organizations or communities offer trauma-informed services, it promotes well-being among survivors, improves skills among those who receive training, and increases collaboration. However, these changes come with resistance. The barriers include a lack of communication, leadership buy-in, competing priorities, financial constraints, lack of perceived relevance, inflexible policies, and procedures, and fears (Huo et al., 2023). These roadblocks will need to be addressed prior to implementation of such a system.

Cultivate Knowledge

Several professions are mentioned along with suggestions for becoming trauma sensitive to their clientele. Add your thoughts here:

- What are practical steps that law enforcement officers can take to increase trauma sensitivity without compromising their primary objectives?
- How could medical providers or medical agencies offer trauma-informed services?
- What further actions could teachers employ in classroom settings to manage their classes yet provide trauma-sensitive teaching?
- Are there other professions that can practice trauma-informed care? How could they do so?

A Flourishing Focus

It may seem obvious that trauma permeates our world. But differing opinions exist regarding its ubiquity. Strike up a conversation with someone about historical trauma, and you will soon hear how someone disagrees that it exists. Some say, "There's no such thing." Others add, "That event never happened." Or start a discussion on rape, and the prevalence of the pervasive myths will shock you. "She wanted it." "The way she dressed was asking for it." Even a discussion about PTSD can cause controversy. We saw an advertisement for a university debate on whether diagnosis is an excuse. Our first thought was, "An excuse for what?" This is a way of thinking about people and the world. Despite a growing understanding of trauma, our community has not yet achieved a trauma-sensitive perspective, and, as a result, we may contribute to someone's trauma.

A change in paradigm is necessary, not just for mental health providers, but for all helpers, and the rest of the world. But this shift is hard and comes with various roadblocks. Like viewing things through a kaleidoscope, we perceive the world according to our histories and expectations. But when we turn the tool a different way, we find variegations of what we thought existed. Moving to a trauma-sensitive outlook requires us to see the world through a different lens. Rather than thinking of people in a derogatory manner, trauma training leads us to understanding why people say what they do and act in certain ways. We learn to listen in a non-judgmental way to the story that unfolds. Our role is not to decipher the truth, but to attune to the person's need for sharing their narrative. In a sense, we become explorers instead of investigators, searching for clues about what happened, how that affects an individual, their relationships, and community, and what the path of the future may be. Some may assume the person with trauma is seeking attention. Perhaps that is true. But, if so, that does not negate their experience, nor their need for human connection. After all, as human beings, we all need people who hear our voices. That is not a negative characteristic that we should dismiss as despised. Instead, we should celebrate that one requests such help.

When asked to change worldviews, people ignore or deny a new way of thinking. They may even attack it, especially if it requires a large amount of time or resources. Some do not realize why such alterations are necessary. This means that we emphasize the burdens of the current systems of care and the profitability of change.

Communities and individuals are the agents of restoration. This view requires awareness, advocacy, and securing opportunities to develop policies, regulations, and preventive techniques, retribution, and holding perpetrators accountable to individuals and the community. Change can only occur when people, leaders, and stakeholders understand the importance of such renovation.

Perhaps sharing the prevalence of trauma in American lives is vital. Almost 60% of adults in the U.S. report experiencing at least one type of childhood trauma (Bethell et al., 2017; Merrick et al., 2019). This means that most Americans entering healthcare and school systems will be on high alert, untrusting, less likely to follow directions, have poor concentration and poor memory skills, and may be less cooperative. This may frustrate healthcare workers and educators. Trauma from assault occurs to 44% of all women and assault occurs in 27% of men (Farahi & McEachern, 2021; Thomas & Kopel, 2023). Many people do not report rape because of their fear of the criminal justice system and the treatment they will receive (Rich, 2019). When they do contact police or legal advocates, they may withhold information, arrive late, tell inaccurate information, be reluctant to participate, have poor eye contact, or be disrespectful. Trauma may be the reason. In America, 20% of police calls for service involve either a mental health or substance use crisis. Even though most traumatized people are not violent, in such a situation, they are more likely to be killed by the police. Approximately 25% of police shooting deaths occur during a mental health crisis (Smith, 2023). The victim may be anxious, uncooperative, shaky, and paranoid, leading an officer to believe they are hiding something or guilty of a criminal offense. These may be signs of trauma. However, when workers are not trained to be traumainformed, the lack of recognition of trauma symptoms may lead them to take actions that result in mismanagement of the situation and lead to dire results. These events can also cause secondary trauma to workers without sufficient support or education.

Sparking a Vision

Communities and individuals are the agents of restoration. This view requires awareness, advocacy, and securing opportunities to develop policies, regulations, and laws to prevent, provide retribution, and rehabilitate those who perpetrate individuals and the community (Ginwright, 2018). Changing paradigm requires an enormous investment of energy, time, resources, finances, and requires collaboration between trauma experts and others. Transforming communities into effective trauma-informed caring environments requires a multilayered approach that addresses systemic and orga-nizational policies, procedures, training, and practical implementation. This change will only be effective when a multifaceted research process ensues (Stillerman et al., 2023). Implementation requires focusing on assets that drive communities to highlight strengths rather than deficits. People are more than their experiences, their diagnosis, or character defaults (Ginwright, 2018).

Helping those invested realize they can be agents of hope when they view traumatic experiences as a collective experience instead of an individual experience changes the world. A colleague describes how her paradigm shifted.

> On a trip to Rwanda to explore recovery efforts from the genocide event in 1994, I witnessed this type of posttraumatic growth as a woman shared her story of survival and revealed her scars from repeated machete strikes while seated next to her perpetrator. They lived and worked together in a reconcili-ation village, which they helped build. Seeing her growth, forgiveness, and acceptance of the traumatic events was astonishing. I learned the South African term *ubuntu* in Rwanda, meaning that we find goodness in being human through collective interdependence and service to others.
>
> When I returned home, I could not stop thinking about this woman, how she lived in the same village with her perpetrator, called him friend, and how they worked together to restore their community. I wondered what I could do, or my community, to move toward such a model of resilience (Figure 9.2).

Assuming responsibility for healing empowers us to explore innovative futures. It is possible to become such a community as Johnson City, Tennessee, who developed their System of Care after receiving a grant in 2013 for crime reduction. This funding was granted for three years, but the community programs developed by Becky Haas and her team were so successful, the community determined they needed to continue their efforts to involve more organizations and local systems in building systems of care for their region (Campbell, 2020). Building a trauma-informed system provided benefits beyond what the community imagined. The System of Care model provided a common language, multiple points of contact, cultural change, and empowered peo-ple. In providing community training, collective resilience increased (Haas & Clements, 2019). Johnson City shows when trauma care can be consistent throughout the com-munity, people are less likely to be re-traumatized, and the community experiences

A Flourishing Focus

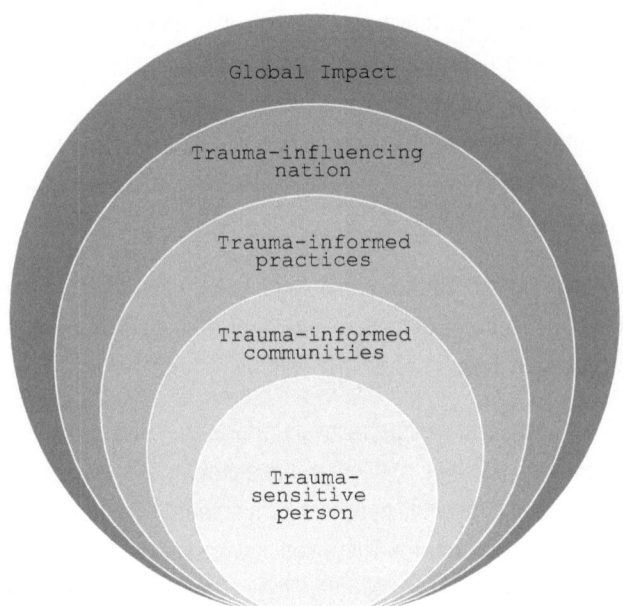

FIGURE 9.2 Global Impact.

better health and mental health outcomes (Haas & Clements, 2019). As we move to becoming trauma-informed communities, what does that mean? What needs to shift in our perspectives?

Tending Your Technique

You are a leader in your professional community and are asked to provide training in trauma competency for your profession. Create a presentation that includes ten slides that define competency and lists specific training, or skills needed.

Becoming a Resilient Society

Developing resilient communities and professionals requires intentionality. As we reflect on the trauma that individuals, families, and communities experience, we must stop and ask what we have learned from those situations. Just as the inner rings of a tree tell its age, they also reveal the tree's history, whether the year was wet or dry, cooler, or hotter. The rings can reveal information about fires or inset outbreaks, or the quality of the wood fiber. This science, dendrochronology, tells us about forests and how those have made it through the worst times and yet provided the best resources for plants, animals, and humans (Steel et al., 2024).

Just as trees survive, and their rings reveal the tale, so our communities have a shared story. While trauma may happen to an individual, we bear responsibility for how we excuse those who wounded the person, and how we treat the traumatized individual. When crises or disasters arrive, and though we wish they would not, they become opportunities to use our collective strength and knowledge. It also means that we discover our vulnerabilities and work to improve those (Imperiale & Vanclay, 2021). We prepare for future crises and disasters, understanding they will inevitably return, despite our best efforts to prevent them. For example, Wilkes-Barre, Pennsylvania, learned a hard lesson when Hurricane Agnes sent torrential rains into the area, flooding the Susquehanna River and much of the area in 1972. Afterward, the U.S. Army Corps of Engineers recognized this weakness and built a levee system, and enhanced it in 1996 (Frantz, 2012). Unfortunately, all towns resting on the beautiful river were at risk, but not all developed a levee system, so when Hurricane Irene arrived in 2012, more towns were devastated, receiving anywhere from 6 inches to 6 feet of water. The governor declared a state of emergency (Meyer, 2012). While the cities with levees were protected, those without levees lost businesses and homes. Afterward, teams met for city planning to discuss how to prevent such loss again. Our vulnerabilities go beyond physical property and material goods. They include our psychological susceptibilities to fear, loss of community connection, loss of peace, and exposure to the negative impact of disaster (Collodi et al., 2021; Rania et al., 2019).

In resilient societies, we recognize that trauma, crises, and disaster not only affect an individual but also impairs the community's well-being when it affects physical and mental health, increases the cost and labor of care, affects cultural practices and beliefs, livelihoods, a community's infrastructure, housing, or capability to afford housing, quality of the environment, and natural resources (Imperiale & Vanclay, 2021). With this cognizance comes the understanding of our joint capacities when we work together. While disaster requires collaboration, times of peace should invite us to plan and celebrate together, to harness our resources, evaluate our progress, and attend to our most vulnerable populations. This interaction only occurs when we develop communities of empathy with a shared perception of needs, desires to enhance well-being, and an attitude of social responsibility. With this, we can create a sustainable culture of resilience wherein we teach one another, and our children,

A Flourishing Focus

the values, beliefs, knowledge, and tools needed. Such a change must be multidimensional, horizontal, and vertical, including all who desire a voice. But it begins with a single person saying, "I believe this is important. Together, we can do this."

Gather Self-Awareness

- How can an organization or community change to becoming trauma-responsive?
- Name the most common barriers faced in changing to a trauma-informed approach.
- What action steps can a community take to develop a trauma-informed system of care?

Chapter Summary

This chapter discussed the dilemma of those who deny the prevalence of trauma and its effect on society. That a change in paradigm is necessary is no surprise, not just for mental health providers, but for all helpers, and the rest of the world. It means moving from "What is wrong with you?" to asking "What happened to you?" The chapter discussed the importance of communities and individuals as agents of restoration, requiring awareness, advocacy, and securing opportunities to develop policies, regulations, and interventions. The discussion included the cost of moving to a different worldview, which requires an enormous investment of energy, time, resources, finances, and requires collaboration between trauma experts and others. Transforming communities into effective trauma-informed caring environments requires a multilayered approach that addresses systemic and organizational policies, procedures, training, and practical implementation. The process of developing a trauma-informed community involves engaging counselors, educators, judges, and other community leaders to be advocates who offer to speak on behalf of creating such a system. These advocates should use a common language with the universal understanding, empowering everyone they encounter to create organizational and community cultural change.

An exploration of trauma competency ensued, including what makes an effective worker, and the specific competencies for counselors who desire to engage in trauma work. Unfortunately, few graduate programs prepare students for trauma-informed counseling and so they must seek additional education upon graduation to become competent. Recommendations for provided for those who desire to continue in gaining expertise.

Finally, the chapter concludes with a discussion of how to create resilient societies, and how trauma, crises, and disaster not only affect an individual but also impair the community's well-being when it affects physical and mental health, increasing the cost and labor of care, affects cultural practices and beliefs, livelihoods, a community's infrastructure, housing, or capability to afford housing, quality of the environment, and natural resources. With this cognizance comes the understanding of our joint capacities when we work together. While disaster requires collaboration, times of peace should invite us to plan and celebrate together, to harness our resources, evaluate our progress, and attend to our most vulnerable populations. This interaction only occurs when we develop communities of empathy with a shared perception of needs, desires to enhance wellbeing, and an attitude of social responsibility.

Chapter Review

Please respond to the following questions:

1. What are the challenges faced by individuals with trauma when interacting with community businesses and agencies?
2. What are the characteristics of effective trauma workers?
3. What suggestions are offered for building resilient communities?
4. How has your motivation shifted throughout the readings?
5. What is your next step in becoming a trauma worker?

Key Term Assessment

Review the following terms and try to explain each concept.

- Paradigm
- Trauma-informed community
- Trauma competency
- Resilience communities

Chapter Summary

Resources

The following resources may be helpful. At the time of this writing, they were accessible through the links provided.

- CPTSD Foundation offers help for healing and trauma recovery through offering therapy networks, coaching, legal services, and research.
- Guidelines on Trauma Competencies for Education Approved by APA Council of Representatives. https://www.apa.org/ed/resources/trauma-competencies-training.pdf
- National Institute for the Clinical Application of Behavioral Medicine (NICABM) offers training and education on trauma, treatments for trauma, and research.
- The National Child Traumatic Stress Network (NCTSN). For help with children, adolescents, and families, NCTSN offers information, training, and other resources of support.
- U.S. Department of Veterans Affairs. PTSD: National Center for PTSD. This site is the world's leading research and educational center on PTSD. It offers practical advice, access to resources, and helpful information about traumatic stress disorders.

References

Albrink, L. G. (2023). Trauma-informed legal advocacy. *Wake Forest Journal of Law & Policy, 13,* 67–102. https://heinonline.org/HOL/P?h=hein.journals/wfjlapo13&i=80

American Psychological Association. (2015). *Guidelines on trauma competencies for education and training.* American Psychological Association.

Baranowsky, A. B. (2019, June 16). *Trauma therapists' 11 BEST practices.* Traumatology Institute.

Bethell, C., Davis, M., Gombojav, N., Stumbo, S., & Powers, K. (2017). Issue brief: A national and across state profile on adverse childhood experiences among children and possibilities to heal and thrive. *The Child & Adolescent Health Measurement Initiative.* https://www.cahmi.org/docs/default-source/resources/issue-brief-a-national-and-across-state-profile-on-adverse-childhood-experiences-among-children-and-possibilities-to-heal-and-thrive-(2017)b0dbc65c3a0944a9854e1fb307d8d0fd.pdf?sfvrsn=95d28208_0

Bosk, E. A., Williams-Butler, A., Ruisard, D., & MacKenzie, M. J. (2020). Frontline staff characteristics and capacity for trauma-informed care: Implications for the child welfare workforce. *Child Abuse & Neglect, 110*(Pt 3), 104536. https://doi.org/10.1016/j.chiabu.2020.104536

Campbell, B. (2020, July 5). *Johnson City's trauma informed system of care is model for the country.* Johnson City Press. https://www.johnsoncitypress.com/johnson-citys-trauma-informed-system-of-care-is-model-for-the-country/article_b6bbddcd-b3fc-5b31-b889-1c0527d6fe16.html

Chin, B., Amin, Q., Hernandez, N., Wright, D.-D., Awan, M. U., Plumley, D., Zito, T., & Elkbuli, A. (2024). Evaluating the effectiveness of trauma-informed care frameworks in provider education and the care of traumatized patients. *Journal of Surgical Research, 296,* 621–635. https://doi.org/10.1016/j.jss.2024.01.042

Clements, A., Haas, B., Cyphers, N. A., Hoots, V., & Barnet, J. (2020). Creating a communitywide system of trauma-informed care. *Progress in Community Health Partnerships: Research, Education, and Action, 14*(4), 499–507. https://doi.org/10.1353/cpr.2020.0055

Collodi, J., Pelling, M., Fraser, A., Borie, M., & Di Vicenz, S. (2021). How do you build back better so no one is left behind? Lessons from Sint Maarten, Dutch Caribbean, following Hurricane Irma. *Disasters, 45*(1), 202–223. https://doi.org/10.1111/disa.12423

Cook, J. M., & Newman, E. (2017). Training in trauma: New Haven Consensus Conference conclusions on core competencies. In S. N. Gold (Ed.), *APA handbook of trauma psychology: Foundations in knowledge* (pp. 145–157). American Psychological Association. https://doi.org/10.1037/0000019-009

Cook, J. M., Newman, E., & Simiola, V. (2019). Trauma training: Competencies, initiatives, and resources. *Psychotherapy, 56*(3), 409–421. https://doi.org/10.1037/pst0000233

Cook, J. M., Newman, E., & The New Haven Trauma Competency Group. (2014). A consensus statement on trauma mental health: The New Haven Competency Conference process and major findings. *Psychological Trauma: Theory, Research, Practice, and Policy, 6*(4), 300–307. https://doi.org/10.1037/a0036747

Elisseou, S., Shamaskin-Garrowway, A., Kopstick, A. J., Potter, J., Weil, A., Gundacker, C., & Moreland-Capuia, A. (2024). Leading organizations from burnout to trauma-informed resilience: A vital paradigm shift. *The Permanente Journal, 28*(1), 198–205. https://www.thepermanentejournal.org/doi/pdf/10.7812/TPP/23.110

Farahi, N., & McEachern, M. (2021). Sexual assault of women. *American Family Physician, 103*(3), 168–176. https://www.aafp.org/pubs/afp/issues/2021/0201/p168.html

Foltz, R., Kaeley, A., Kupchan, J., Mills, A., Murray, K., Pope, A., Rahman, H., & Rubright, C. (2023). Trauma-informed care? Identifying training deficits in accredited doctoral programs. *Psychological Trauma: Theory, Research, Practice, and Policy, 15*(7), 1188–1193. https://doi.org/10.10037/tra0001461

Frantz, J. (2012, September 16). Tropical Storm Lee's lasting impact: West Pittston residents look for chance to make the town 'great again'. *PENN LIVE Patriot News.* https://www.pennlive.com/midstate/2012/09/tropical_storm_lees_lasting_im_7.html

Gentry, J. E., Baranowsky, A. B., & Rhoton, R. (2017). Trauma competency: An active ingredient approach to treating posttraumatic stress disorder. *Journal of Counseling & Development, 95*(3), 245–366. https://aztrauma.org/wp-content/uploads/2018/01/Trauma-Competency-JCD.pdf

Ginwright, S. (2018, May 31). *The future of healing: Shifting from trauma informed care to healing centered engagement.* https://ginwright.medium.com/the-future-of-healing-shifting-from-trauma-informed-care-to-healing-centered-engagement-634f557ce69c

Haas, B., & Clements, A. D. (2019). *Building a trauma informed system of care.* State of Tennessee Department of Children's Services. https://www.tn.gov/content/dam/tn/dcs/documents/health/aces/building-strong-brains-tn/Building%20a%20Trauma%20Informed%20System%20of%20Care%20Toolkit.pdf

Henning, J. A., Brand, B., & Courtois, C. A. (2022). Graduate training and certification in trauma treatment for clinical practitioners. *Training and Education in Professional Psychology, 16*(4), 362–375.

Huo, Y., Couzner, L., Windsor, T., Laver, K., Dissanayaka, N. N., & Cations, M. (2023). Barriers and enablers for the implementation of trauma-informed care in healthcare settings: A systematic review. *Implementation Science Communications, 4*(49). https://doi.org/10.1186/s43058-023-00428-0

Imperiale, A. J., & Vanclay, F. (2021). Conceptualizing community resilience and the social dimensions of risk to overcome barriers to disaster risk reduction and sustainable development. *Sustainable Development, 29*(5), 891–905, https://doi.org/10.1002/sd.2182

Knight, C. (2018). Trauma-informed supervision: Historical antecedents, current practice, and future directions. *The Clinical Supervisor, 37*(1), 7–37. https://doi.org/10.1080/07325223.2017.1413607

Levinson, W., Gorawara-Bhat, R., & Lamb, J. (2000). A study of patient clues and physician responses in primary care and surgical settings. *Journal of the American Medical Association, 284*(8), 1021–1027. https://doi.org/10.1001/jama.284.8.1021

Lewis, C., Raisanen, L., Bisson, J. I., Jones, I., & Zammit, S. (2018). Trauma exposure and undetected posttraumatic stress disorder among adults with a mental disorder. *Depression and Anxiety, 35*(2), 178–184. https://doi.org/10.1002/da.22707

Lorey, K., & Fegert, J. M. (2022). Incorporating mental health literacy and trauma-informed law enforcement: A participative survey on police officers' attitudes and knowledge concerning mental disorders, traumatization, and trauma sensitivity. *Psychological Trauma: Theory, Research, Practice, and Policy, 14*(2), 218–228. https://doi.org/10.1037/tra0001067

Ludick, M., & Figley, C. R. (2017). Toward a mechanism for secondary trauma induction and reduction: Reimagining a theory of secondary traumatic stress. *Traumatology, 23*(1), 112–123. https://doi.org/10.1037/trm0000096

Mathew, S., Qiao, B., & Kaszynski, E. (2023). Training counselors to provide trauma informed care: CACREP-accredited program survey. *International Journal for Multidisciplinary Research*, *5*(4), 1–5.

Melegkovits, E., Blumberg, J., Dixon, E., Ehntholt, K., Gillard, J., Kayal, H., Kember, T., Ottisova, L., Walsh, E., Wood, M., Gafoor, R., Brewin, C., Billings, J., Robertson, M., & Bloomfield, M. (2023). The effectiveness of trauma-focused psychotherapy for complex posttraumatic stress disorder: A retrospective study. *European Psychiatry*, *66*(1), e4, 1–9.

Merrick, M. T., Ford, D. C., Ports, K. A., Guinn, A. S., Chen, J., Klevens, J., Metzler, M., Jones, C. M., Simon, T. R., Daniel, V. M., Ottley, P., & Mercy, J. A. (2019). Estimated proportion of adult health problems attributable to adverse childhood experiences and implications for prevention—25 States, 2015–2017. *Morbidity and Mortality Weekly Report*, *68*(44), 999–1005. https://doi.org/10.15585/mmwr.mm6844e1

Meyer, J. (2012, September 7). The unforgettable flood. *WNEP 16 The News Station*. https://www.wnep.com/article/news/local/bradford-county/the-unforgetable-flood/523-4a4c5c78-d914-4b68-ab3c-c448997b9c1a

Miller, B., & Sprang, G. (2017). A components-based practice and supervision model for reducing compassion fatigue by affecting clinician experience. *Traumatology*, *23*(2), 153–164. https://doi.org/10.1037/trm0000058

Morton, B. M. (2022). Trauma-informed school practices: Creating positive classroom culture. *Middle School Journal*, *53*(4), 20–27. https://doi.org/10.1080/00940771.2022.2096817

Norrish, J., & Brunzell, T. (2023). How is trauma-informed education implemented within classrooms? A synthesis of trauma-informed education programs. *Australian Journal of Teacher Education*, *48*(3), 6. https://doi.org/10.14221/1835-517X.6159

Pohl, S., Larsen, R., & McCormick, S. (2021, November 29). Five ways to practice trauma-informed leadership. *Accelerate: Learning Community*. https://accelerate.uofuhealth.utah.edu/leadership/five-ways-to-practice-trauma-informed-leadership

Rania, N., Coppola, I., Martorana, F., & Migliorini, L. (2019). The collapse of the Morandi Bridge in Genoa on 14 August 2018: A collective traumatic event and its emotional impact linked to the place and loss of a symbol. *Sustainability*, *11*(23), 6822. https://doi.org/10.3390/su11236822

Ray, S. L., Wong, C., White, D., & Heaslip, K. (2013). Compassion satisfaction, compassion fatigue, work life conditions, and burnout among frontline mental health care professionals. *Traumatology*, *19*(4), 255–267. https://doi.org/10.1177/1534765612471144

Rich, K. (2019). Trauma-informed police responses to rape victims. *Journal of Aggression, Maltreatment & Trauma*, *28*(4), 463–480. https://doi.org/10.1080/10926771.2018.1540448

Singer, P. (2024). Toward a more trauma-informed church: Equipping faith communities to prevent and respond to abuse. *Currents in Theology and Mission*, *51*(1), 62–76.

References

Smith, C. M. (2023). *Trauma-informed criminal justice*. https://www.rstreet.org/wp-content/uploads/2023/08/FINAL-trauma-informed-CJ-08-23.pdf

Steel, E. A., Hinckley, T. M., Richards, W. H., & D'Amore, D. V. (2024). Chapter 3 – Forests then and now: Managing for ecosystem benefits, services to humans, and healthy forests across scales. In S. G. McNulty (Ed.), *Future forests: Mitigation and adaptation to climate* change (pp. 49–64). https://doi.org/10.1016/B978-0-323-90430-8.00009-5

Stillerman, A., Altman, L., Peña, G., Cua, G., Goben, A., Walden, A., & Atkins, M. (2023). Advancing trauma-informed care in hospitals: The time is now. *The Permanente Journal, 27*, 16–20. https://doi.org/10.7812/TPP/22.081

Substance Abuse and Mental Health Services Administration (SAMHSA). (2014). *SAMHSA's concept of trauma and guidance for a trauma-informed approach* [pdf file]. Substance Abuse and Mental Health Services Administration.

Substance Abuse and Mental Health Services Administration (SAMHSA). (2024). *Trauma training for criminal justice professionals*. https://www.samhsa.gov/gains-center/trauma-training-criminal-justice-professionals

Taylor, C. L. (2016). Relationships among resilience, trauma scientific knowledge, perceived competence to treat and emotional competence toward complex trauma cases among mental health trainees [Dissertation, University of Kansas].

Thomas, J. C., & Kopel, J. (2023). Male victims of sexual assault: A review of the literature. *Behavioral Sciences, 13*(4), 304. https://doi.org/10.3390/bs13040304

Trzeciak, S., & Mazzarelli, A. (2019). *Compassionomics: The revolutionary scientific evidence that caring makes a difference*. Studer Group.

Van der Merwe, A., & Hunt, X. (2019). Secondary trauma among trauma researchers: Lessons from the field. *Psychological Trauma: Theory, Research, Practice, and Policy, 11*(1), 10–18. https://doi.org/10.1037/tra0000414

Weiss, R., Vittinghoff, E., Fang, M. C., Cimino, J. E. W., Chasteen, K. A., Arnold, R. M., Auerbach, A. D., & Anderson, W. G. (2017). Associations of physician empathy with patient anxiety and ratings of communication in hospital admission encounters. *Journal of Hospital Medicine, 12*(10), 805–810. https://doi.org/10.12788/jhm.2828

Wexler, E. (2024). *Trauma-informed policing: A special set to tools for law enforcement* [presentation]. https://health.maryland.gov/bha/Documents/Trauma-Informed%20Policing%20-%20Betsy%20Wexler.pdf

Index

Page numbers in *italics* denote figures; page numbers in **bold** denote tables